How to Overcome Snoring

(With Warm Fuzzies
in Recovery and Ecstasy)

By Ronald Alan Duskis, D.C., B.A. Zoology, B.A. Theology

toExcel

San Jose New York Lincoln Shanghai

**How to Overcome Snoring
(With warm Fuzzies in Recovery and Ecstasy)**

Published by toExcel
an imprint of iUniverse.com, Inc.

For information address:
iUniverse.com, Inc.
620 North 48th Street
Suite 201
Lincoln, NE 68504-3467
www.iuniverse.com

ISBN: 0-595-00473-3

Printed in the United States of America

TABLE OF CONTENTS

About the Author

Dr. Ronald Alan Duskis, has worked in the profession of Chiropractor for 18 years and has been a Massage Therapist for 22 years. He holds a B.A. in Zoology and a B.A. in Theology. Ron is the author of two other books: <u>Back to Health</u> and <u>Odors From Head to Toe:</u>, both of which are available upon request. Ron makes his home in Fort Collins, Colorado with his lovely wife, Pina and two daughters.

About the Editor

Elaine Tregenza Burritt has a Master's degree in Library Science and has worked in libraries for 17 years. She is an avid reader, writer, and enjoys reviewing other's writings. Elaine also resides in Fort Collins with her husband, Don, and kitty, Misha.

DEDICATION

I wish to dedicate this book to all people who have suffered seconds, minutes, hours, weeks, months, or years with personal snoring or another person's or pet's snoring! Someday, when the battle to overcome snoring is won, we veterans shall look back at our suffering as a sacrifice of much needed sleep for our loved ones who, "could not help it, " or , "did not know they were snoring, keeping us up. " We then will be glad that this plague is over!

ACKNOWLEDGEMENTS

I want to thank all the people who gave me their testimonials so that thousands, if not millions of people, can live a better, more restful night.

A special thanks goes to my wife, Pina, and my two daughters, Chrissy and Charissa, for sacrificing many hours while I sat at the computer working on this book.

Thanks to my wife, I learned that I too would snore at night which stirred me to action to find preventions, helps, and cures in order not to bother her sleep at night.

Thanks also goes to my daughter, Chrissy, who has always been there for me encouraging me to do the jobs, such as this one, that I enjoy most.

And a big thanks goes also to my ten year old daughter, Charissa, who spent hours at the library with me encouraging me to research more and more information on this subject.

A WORD FROM THE EDITOR

I really did not know very much about the subject of snoring when Ron asked me to be his editor. I, of course, am NOT a snorer (not yet, anyway); although, I am familiar with the state of snoring from sharing motel rooms with both of my parents, and occasionally my husband (with his poor chronically stuffed up nose) snores. But, in reading through the manuscript, I have learned a lot! This book is crammed full of funny stories, helpful suggestions, and information about snoring and its causes and effects. As a librarian, I can see that Dr. Duskis has thoroughly researched his subject matter and compiled useful information from many sources.

Let me share my snoring story with you: "The loudest snoring I ever heard was on a camping trip in Arizona. My girlfriend invited me to go with her parents and uncle, warning me ahead of time that her family were extremely vocal snorers. She strongly suggested that I bring along earplugs. I can usually sleep through just about anything; however, the noises reverberated throughout the trailer, and I was forced to use some earplugs to block out the snoring and get some sleep myself."

Well, read on to the useful and entertaining book that Dr. Duskis has authored. And Snore No More!

Elaine T. Burritt

PREFACE FROM THE AUTHOR

Snoring has probably bothered people since the beginning of time. Literally millions of people snore. Today, thanks to modern Medicine and all of the alternative healing arts, people need to snore no more! There are ways to help the snorer, prevent the snoring, and even to cure the snoring. I have just completed this book that shows you how!

From all of the research that has been done on snoring, the main problem that appears to cause the snoring is found in either the nose or back of the mouth or both. Sometimes the person only has a deviated nasal septum, and an operation can remove this cause of the snoring. And sometimes the person who snores may have enlarged and/or inflamed tissues in the back of the mouth that flutter when the snorer breathes air inward. In the latter case, removing the enlarged tissue or the inflammation can remove these causes of the snoring. Allergies can inflame the nasal and back of the mouth regions that will result in a snore. By the healing of the allergy involved, the snoring is reduced or eliminated. Another example is found in overweight people. Here, the tissues enlarge throughout the body, including the back of the mouth. Another example is the smoker who irritates or inflames the back of his/her mouth which results in snoring. Other reasons include psychological, exercise abuse, eating abuse, and drinking abuse.

Even the nervous system can be involved in the production of the snore. If the nervous system is not working right to the nasal and/or back of the mouth regions, inflammations may result that lead to snoring. I have found in my own personal life that snoring is reduced by working on my neck vertebrae and the associated muscles.

This book includes alternative methods that have helped, prevented, and/or cured snoring. For example, many times a snore would not take place unless the snorer slept with the mouth open. There are ways to help train the snorer on how to keep his/her mouth closed. This would prevent the back of the mouth from drying out which would prevent greater flutter of the parts in the back of the mouth. And there is another book that explains how to oil, with vegetable oil of a certain kind, the nasal and back of the mouth regions to prevent and possibly even eliminate the snoring for the night.

Over twenty chapters cover so much material on snoring that the reader will probably find something to use to have a good night's sleep. There is even a section on animals that snore! Happy reading and no more snoring!

Dr. Ronald Alan Duskis

On the next page is the snoring questionnaire that may be filled out by any reader who would like to participate in any future edition of this snoring book. Please do not feel that it is too late to fill this out no matter what date you are reading this book, because I plan on updating my book every year. Therefore, please fill it out today, if you would be so kind. You will find some testimonials in this book, and I hope to include even more in the next edition. You will probably help many people here in America get a good night's sleep if you do it now! Thank you all in advance for your help in my book updates!

THE SNORING QUESTIONNAIRE

     I the undersigned understand that Ronald Alan Duskis is gathering real life experiences and knowledge dealing with snoring. The following are my experiences or knowledge dealing with this subject that may be used in any of his literature or publications in full or part anytime with my complete consent and blessing in his using it without any money ever to be given to me or anyone else.

     Date_____

     Signed_____

     Print your name_____
     Address_____
     Phone number_____

1. Do you know of any funny stories about snoring?_____
_____
_____.

2. How do you prevent snoring? _____
_____

3 .   H o w   d o   y o u   h e l p   o v e r c o m e   s n o r i n g ?
_____
_____.

4 .   H o w   d o   y o u   c u r e   o r   e l i m i n a t e   s n o r i n g ?
_____

5. How does snoring effect social life?:
   A. In marriage_____
_____.
   B. In room-mate situations:_____
_____.
   C. Between brothers and sisters:_____
_____.
   D. Between parents and children:_____
_____.
   E. Any other situations socially:_____
_____.

6. How do or did you cope with any of the situations listed in number 5 above?:_____
_____
_____.

7. What do you think and/or feel about while you are near another person snoring? Check off those that apply below:
A. Person is tired_____ B. Person is ill_____
C. Person is stressed out_____ D. Person needs pity_____

E. Person is selfish_____   F. Person does not care about you___   G. Any other comment_____

_____.

8. Do you know if you personally snore?_____. What do you think and/or feel about your own snoring?_____
_____. What do you feel others are thinking or feeling about you?

_____.

9. Any other comments_____
_____
_____.

Please mention whether I can use your full name or just your initials in my quoting you in my literature_____.   Also may I use your full address or just your city and state:_____.
If you leave these two last answers blank then it gives me permission to only use your initials with a city and state.

_____

To all people participating in my writing on snoring:

Thank you for participating in one of the most needful writings in the decade of the 90s. Your help will be greatly appreciated by the many people who suffer at night having to listen to other people snoring. Your help will possibly reach not only thousands, but hopefully millions, in the months and years to come. So please take your time in filling out the page that has space for your experiences and/or knowledge dealing with this subject. Copy that page if you need more room or if you wish to give some copies to your friends so they too can participate. And please do not forget to fill in all signature spaces with your signature; and answer any questions that pertain to you on the bottom of that page from numbers 1 through 5 (number 5 can be a name title like Dr. to be included or it can be that you want your business name and your title to be included in the writing of this book). Please then return the page(s) to me as soon as possible so that your writing may be included in the upcoming edition. It is never to late to send in your testimonial as new editions should be made periodically. Once again, thank you for your help and participation!

Remember, that by participating, you can help your fellow man not only get a good night sleep; but you may save yourself from having to be with a sleepy friend or business associate who needs to read your message in this book to deal vitally with you! If enough people just read this book, you and others will experience a world different from what we find today where we all will feel wide awake and more desirous to love and serve each other! Also, the fear of not knowing whether the person you are talking to got you message due to a tired mind from a lack of sleep will be gone!

And who knows just how many new friends and relationships can be attracted to you because these people are alert enough in mind to acknowledge, appreciate, and realize you. Many readers will be thankful to you for having saved them from the snoring of mates, room mates, relatives, friends, etc.! These readers have wanted to know answers to overcoming snoring but did not know a book to find the answers in! Now you can help!

So give to your fellow man your best experiences and/or knowledge dealing with overcoming snoring. I thank you for your help in accomplishing the completion of this coming edition!

Thank you again for your kindness in sharing,

May 15, 1991
Date Signed

Ronald Alan Duskis
2800 Calendar Court
Fort Collins, Colorado 80526

To all Doctors and others desiring to participate in this project:

I understand that Ronald Alan Duskis is gathering real life experiences and knowledge dealing with snoring. The following are my experiences or knowledge dealing with this subject that may be used in any of his literature or publications in full or part anytime with my complete consent and blessing in his using it without any money ever to be given to me or anyone else.

Signed_____Date_____
Print Your Name_____
Address_____
Phone Number_____

_____
_____
_____
_____
_____
_____
_____
_____
_____
_____
_____
_____
_____
_____
_____
_____
_____
_____
_____
_____
_____
_____
_____
_____
_____
_____
_____
_____
_____
_____
_____

Signed_____Date_____
Place your signature in the following desired:
1. I want my name and address in your printing_____.
2. I only want my name printed in your work_____.
3. I only want my initials and city and state_____.
4. I definitely want my phone number listed_____.
5. Special further instructions as needed_____
_____.

SNORING: A PSYCHOTHERAPIST'S VIEWPOINT

Written by Douglas D. Settles, M. A., a psychotherapist who operates Choices: a Center for Emotional and Spiritual Growth in Fort Collins, Colorado.

It was surprising to me when Dr. Duskis asked me to contribute to his book on snoring. What would a psychotherapist know about snoring? I thought hard about whether I had ever had a client of mine that had come to me expressly to get rid of the psychological cause of snoring and if so, what was the effect of the therapy. In all honesty, I had to admit I have never had a client come in specifically for the symptom of snoring! So then, why am I writing this introduction?

I initially said I would write this because of my respect for Dr. Duskis. I told him, "Sure, I'll do it. Why don't you let me read your book and I'll see what I can do." Once I read this great book on snoring, I was absolutely amazed at the similarities of what I do in my office with psychotherapy with my clients and what Dr. Duskis conveyed in his book. In fact, I believe that a psychological/spiritual introduction is just what this book needs to complete the picture of what snoring is all about.

The Body Never Lies

A belief system that is held by some members of the therapy professions (myself included) is that indeed the body never lies. When something is going on with the body, it is trying to tell the individual that something is wrong with his/her lifestyle, life choices, or the path that the person is on. "Something is wrong" and needs to be fixed.

The only problem that I have found with this belief system is learning the language of the body. Sometimes it is like I am speaking English and it is the only language that I know and the body is speaking ancient Latin or some equally foreign or difficult language to understand. <u>What</u> is the body trying to say to me? Such a simple thing as snoring, and the body is trying to tell me something? Yes, I think that is true, and Dr. Duskis does a remarkably good job in conveying just that message to the reader.

The Message

Just what is the message the body is trying to tell us by the snoring? Dr. Duskis tells us that snoring can lead to increased blood pressure, irregular heart functions and sleep apnea. These are all potentially very dangerous physical symptoms to be dealing with. Certainly not a message that should be ignored or overlooked! Snoring can actually be the body's way of communicating to us that we have at least part of our life that is causing some very real danger to us. "Snoring means that a portion of our lives is out of control or unmanageable...(Chapter 3)."

The Specifics

So what is "out of control"? Again, in this book, Dr. Duskis will point out that snoring can have as a root cause being overweight, smoking, having either environmental or food allergies, alcohol or drug abuse, etc.

In the field of therapy, people who do some of the above, can be labelled as addictive personalities and actually be called alcoholic, drug addict, or having an eating disorder. Even less extreme than this, the very use of these substances by some people or even being a few pounds overweight can cause some disastrous results, i.e., snoring and all of the emotional and relationship consequences that are given as examples in this book.

The Task

In the 25 years I have spent in the field of human services, I have helped literally thousands of individuals to overcome and heal addictions such as overeating, alcohol and drugs, and smoking. From this experience, I know it is no easy task. Marcus Boulware states that one needs to just "instruct a snorer how to overcome his bad habits by exercising and self-discipline". He also states that only one of 100,000 snorers needs psychoanalysis. Perhaps it is true that the intensity, length, and expense of psychoanalysis need not be considered for a snorer. I know only a handful of individuals, however, that are addicted to substances like cigarettes, alcohol, drugs, or food that doesn't need some help in overcoming these addictions. Exercise and self-discipline for anyone who needs to lose 50 pounds is virtually an insult. Yet, such programs as Alcoholics Anonymous, Narcotics Anonymous, SmokeEnders, Weight Watchers and a variety of other self-help groups, support groups, or therapy programs have been extremely successful for tens of thousands of individuals.

Choices

The most difficult thing I believe a snorer will be faced with will be the decision to do something about his/her snoring. Such a simple thing as finding out what foods may cause an allergy and then eliminating these specific foods from the diet is actually a very difficult thing for a great deal of people. To have the blood work done, to commit to the cost of the laboratory, and then to find out it may be wheat, chicken, milk, corn, potatoes, or beef can be devastating to the individual if the majority of the diet is composed of these foods. The snorer may well say I will choose to continue to snore if I have to give up my beer, wine, hamburger, or cinnamon roll in the morning.

The choices that the individual makes about his/her snoring will actually have far reaching effects on roommates, spouse, parents, or children that actually have to listen to the snorer! Even though the relationships of the snorer may be threatened, the more serious choice may well be to continue eating a food that may cause the snore or not remove a family pet (cat, dog, or bird) from the house that might cause the allergy. The relationships may not be the ultimate cost of such a decision. High blood pressure and irregular heart functions can have much more serious and perhaps fatal consequences.

What does it take for most people to make such a drastic lifestyle change? Most of the time it takes a crisis of some fair magnitude. A book I once ready many years ago said Human Beings can learn out of love and joy; they, however, insist on learning out of pain and sorrow. How true this is. Most of our greatest lessons and largest growth steps have been because of some significant trauma. Is the mere fact that one snores going to be enough for the individual to find the root cause of the snoring and then to do something about that cause, i.e., make a lifestyle change? Sadly enough, oftentimes it will not be enough. For an alcoholic to lose his/her family, job, and health is oftentimes not enough to stop drinking. Emphysema or lung cancer is often not enough for the smoker to stop smoking. Diabetes, high blood pressure, and asthma may not be enough for the overweight person to choose to do something about the weight problem. Where does snoring fit into such serious business as emphysema, lung cancer, alcoholism, or obesity?

Only the individual person can answer such a significant question and then make the choice.

"To remove the cause is much better than to suffer with the effect." R. Duskis, D.C.

"There it is! Do not ever be too hard on yourself! But do find out the cause for your snoring..." R. Duskis

I believe that all but the most serious student of snoring will find out more on snoring in **this book** than they have ever imagined existed on the subject. I believe the information contained within these pages will help any snorer to overcome their problem. Only the individual can make the choice to do so.

I wish each of you well on your journey to health and happiness by making your **choice**.

INTRODUCTION

The dream to snore no more may now be a reality for many of you according to the writings on this subject! This book is a much needed source of information that may lead anyone to the knowledge, understanding, and wisdom on how to overcome snoring! Some of the information deals with how to prevent snoring; other information deals with only helping the snorer; and still other information deals with the cures of the problem.

It is my deep desire that progress is always made for better treatment of snoring and a better approach on the mental, emotional, and spiritual level. I hope we never go backwards or have to experience a time in history again where an answer to snoring is lacking. For example, Dr. Lipman, M.D. found the following quote in his studies on snoring found in the 1926 Ladies' Home Journal: "Experts are sending us mixed messages about snoring. One thing is for certain, there is no simple answer. If you have a solution, write a book. It can't miss. The world is still waiting...and snoring." (Lipman, Preface, pages viii through ix).

Dr. Lipman, M.D. gives us hope for a better today and tomorrow as will be shown throughout this book: "Today however, snoring has graduated from being regarded as a hopeless nightly nuisance to the level of a legitimate medical problem--as respectable a symptom as back pain or headache. Researchers and clinicians have finally isolated the underlying causes of snoring and are now discovering a variety of realistic treatments for it. These can bring gratifying results to both snorers and snorees." (Lipman, page 16).

And Dr. Lipman, M.D. shows that this was not always the case. We can be very thankful that we are alive in this very end of the twentieth century, and not 20 years ago: "As recently as 20 years ago, for example, the grim prognosis for snorers was summed up by the editor of the British Medical Association's popular monthly Family Doctor: 'I'm not hopeful about a cure for snoring,' he wrote. 'It is unlikely that anyone will come up with anything dramatic or sensational.'" (Lipman, page 16).

Thus, the overall purpose of this book is to fulfill its title which is How to Overcome Snoring With Warm Fuzzies: in Recovery and Ecstasy! That is, to enable the reader to not only recover from the plague of snoring, but to also give him/her the ability to have a good night's sleep! And in the process of recovery and reaching the delightful state of ecstasy, our desire to grow mentally, emotionally, and spiritually needs to be emphasized.

In fact, the reader may want to go directly to the chapter on Warm Fuzzies at the end of this book. This Warm Fuzzies chapter will give the reader the building blocks to a warmer relationship with anyone, whether they are a snorer or not. And it will tell the reader how to work with a snorer while the snorer is in the recovery stage; and then, it will show the reader how to work with the recovered snorer, a period of time I call ecstasy since snoring no longer will tend to put a drag on their hoped for delightful or ecstatic unity!

Yes, it is possible to have an ecstatic or delightful relationship! Certain principles that cause such a life need to be enjoyed and followed to reach that goal. It is possible to reverse a shame-based, unhappy relationship; and to see it convert into a glory-based, ecstatic relationship. Of course the road to this latter relationship takes time and effort, but the rewards are sure and enjoyable! Good health care Professionals need to be consulted in this matter!

These good health care Professionals can guide and direct you to the warm fuzzies that can help you with your life now and forever. These warm fuzzies are ways of life that show whomever we are near that we care, even if they are a snorer. They are not just silly expressions that people might use, but they are ways of life that need to be used. They change people's lives for the better and promote good growth physically, emotionally, mentally, and spiritually.

To this end, this book has been written. This is a unique approach on this subject to the best of my knowledge. All the other books and articles I have read on this subject emphasize overcoming snoring from different angles, but this book is hopefully going to be the first complete book on the subject. My hope is that the reader and I will both develop better character by going through the trial of overcoming snoring in ourselves and in those around us. This is the challenge of this book! So let us get ready to take on responsibilities in our conquering of snoring!

And let us be encouraged to read that even early Doctors have made hope-promoting statements like Dr. Ian Robin in 1968: "Cure is possible in about 50 percent of the cases; 30 percent can be helped by palliative measures; and 20 percent seem hopelessly incurable at the present time." (Boulware, page 33). Note that was as early as 1968, about a quarter of a century ago from the writing of this book. Presently, there is new and exciting information!

But the reader should know that there is probably a lot more information on snoring than he/she realizes. And it is the purpose of this book to put as much of the available information together in simple-to-understand words in a recovery and ecstasy format. That is the major purpose of this book; for you the reader to be able to take as much of the information I have gathered and put it into practice using the proper Professional care.

And on this note of finding the proper Professional care, the book written by Dr. Derek S. Lipman, M.D. gives a notice at the beginning of his book: "**Notice** this book is intended to provide information and entertainment rather than give specific medical advice or advocate one method of treatment over another. To accept medical treatment or undergo surgery is a highly personal decision. That decision should be made only after the treating physician has fully explained every aspect of the recommended therapy or procedure, including the options, risks, and possible complications of such treatments. The author and Rodale Press shall not accept liability or responsibility to any person with respect to loss, injury, or damage caused or alleged to be caused by information contained within this book." (Lipman, **Notice** in front of book). This is to be followed by all readers of this book also as found in the **Notice** since good health care Professionals are needed to offer their services of treatment and surgery for snorers; but personal decision and a number of health care Professional opinions are important before a good decision usually can be reached.

For example, when I was 13 years old, (31 years ago) I broke my nose. The Medical Doctors that first worked on me could not stop the bleeding properly. Thanks to the wisdom that my Dad had, he called Medical Doctor specialists in for more opinions. As I understand the story, he would not let them do anything to me until they all agreed. And once they agreed, my Dad still had to make a personal decision for me whether to proceed. He finally decided to choose one of two ways to correct my bleeding. The decision he made and the work that the Medical Doctors performed turned out to have worked well. I recovered!

My Dad -later told me that there was also another person in the hospital that also had a broken nose from a fight. I was told that they operated on him and he died. Because of that death my Dad felt it would be better to take an alternate course of treatment that had less risk at first; and to do the surgery if necessary. The Medical Doctors found an alternative method of treating me which worked great! I am glad that my Dad and the Medical Doctors had kept up with the latest information in their studies.

The reader is encouraged to go to the Bibliography found at the back of this book, and to go to the library for more current information, and do more research if necessary since it is wise to keep up on the subject. There seems to always be new information that is produced that may help. So be encouraged and continue to read on in this book and other books and literature to learn more about the already found ways and the new ways to conquer snoring!

But I also need to mention something very important that all readers need to follow carefully; it will be up to the reader to read thoroughly this whole book before attempting to follow any of it; and then the reader is obligated to check with his/her Medical Health Professional, such as a personal Medical Doctor or Dentist before attempting to do any of these preventions, helps, or cures for snoring.

I cannot overemphasize the need for Medical Health Professionals to be involved initially and throughout your dealing with this subject on snoring! For example, what if you were allergic to a substance recommended which might injure your health if you took it? "Allergies in the nasal passages are thought to be among the primary factors causing snoring, including industrial air pollution and cigarette smoking. One form of nasal allergy is 'allergic rhinitis.' This condition congests the nasal cavities and often leads to mouth breathing followed by snoring. All mouth breathers do not snore, but a great many of them do." (Boulware, page 61).

And to locate a specialist dealing with sleep disorders in general, the reader can ask their Medical Doctor and ask the American Sleep Disorders Association. Their address is given as, "American Sleep Disorders Association, 604 Second Street Southwest, Rochester, Minnesota, 55902." (Mosley, page 34).

Always go to your Medical Health Professional and other Health Professionals first! This is emphasized by Marcus Boulware, a pioneer snore therapist in 1974, when he stated: "But whatever is done for the patient, he should be under the constant care of the physician until cured or improved." (Boulware, page 50). Amd. "The question of diet in the control of allergies, obesity, and overweight should be the province of the doctor in contradistinction to whatever influence folk cures and remedies may have." (Boulware, page 58).

This is only sound advice if one wants to live a life where he/she loves his/her neighbor as himself/herself. Love for self since snoring many times indicates that a person may be ill; so that helping or curing the snoring will indicate a healthier person. And love for neighbor since the neighbor now can live a healthier life by not being awakened from his much needed sleep required for health. Both of these will be discussed in greater detail throughout this book.

Snoring occurs not only in humans, but also in pets. Looking back at this episode now is rather humorous; but it definitely was not funny in 1960. I remember it well as a child, about 30 years ago. My dog would snore so loudly! I would wake up asking myself in the middle of night when I needed my sleep: "Who's snoring now?" Sometimes my dad would snore and sometimes my two brothers, all three of whom I dared not awaken since I felt they needed their sleep. But when my dog, Kookie, snored, I knew he could sleep most of the day while I was in Jr. High School. I always remember initially laughing when I found out that it was my dog, and I learned to gently urge him out of his snore by saying, "Kookie, Kookie, wake up." Unfortunately, my dog, like a human usually went back into his snore. These repeating situations in my early life led me to begin my studying the subject of snoring in hopes to someday write a book of hope for all people in all generations on the subject. Well, I think that dream has come true with the writing of this book! Here's to a snoreless society now and for all eternity!

At this point it is needed to ask the reader to be patient with their snoring problem and the snoring problem of others around them. The writings that I include in this book claim to prevent, help, and/or cure snoring for many people. I have personally tried the ones I wanted to choose, and have found those to work. There is a great comfort in knowing that these preventions, helps, and cures are available today! And the consolation is that if we all help each other overcome this plague of snoring, the day should come into each of our lives where snoring is eliminated or helped greatly.

And, it is important to counsel about any problems that may be bothering your relationships due to this problem with a good Professional counsellor. A good Professional counsellor may help you get through any uncomfortable emotional or mental stresses: and he/she may help preserve and strengthen your relationship(s).

It is important to note two special chapters at the end of this book that deal with other sleep problems and the concept of dealing with people in a warm fuzzy way. Even these other sleep disorders, other than snoring can be helped, as you can read later in this book: "You can stop losing sleep over your sleeping problems. Persistent sleep disorders that had been accepted as normal consequences of aging are now being researched and diagnosed in the many sleep clinics throughout the nation." (Editors of <u>Prevention</u> Magazine Health Books, page 367).

It is the hope of this book that snoring and other sleep disorders will be viewed differently after either the young or older reader has completed reading and fulfilling necessary sections pertaining to them in this book.

CHAPTER 1: THE HISTORY OF SNORING

The history of snoring probably dates back to the time of Adam and Eve. I am of this opinion since after studying this subject as thoroughly as I have to date, there are so many different reasons or causes for snoring that probably the first man and woman created snored.

In fact, Hoppe feels that all people have an inclination to snore. (Boulware, page 35). And one author says, "Snoring has been with us since time began." (Lipman, page 2). And Dr. Lipman, M.D. says, "Virtually all of us snore now and then. Much of it is mild or occasional snoring--as when a man comes home from a tiring day, falls asleep, and begins to saw away." (Lipman, pages 12 and 13).

The causes of snoring in **all** people will be covered as best as possible in the chapter entitled Chapter 3: "Why snoring? What does it mean? Causes". Also these causes are covered throughout the text of this book.

But right now, let's see historically what well known and not so well known people have been known to snore. There should be no shame in snoring as long as we strive to eliminate the causes of our own personal reasons for snoring which is possible to determine in a good number of cases. Of course to do this, we must search diligently for the cause through **Professional** help and trial and error. Then, we must remove the cause through Professional help and doing our own part to assist.

The aim of this book is to provide historically a gathering of much needed information in hope of seeing people take care of their individual problem of snoring and then to eliminate or lessen it greatly. It would profit the reader to read the articles and books on snoring listed in the Bibliography of my book, and to read new books and articles that can be found in their local library in the future. I just want to let the reader know how happy they and I should be that there is information available for our overcoming this annoying and irritating problem that <u>no one</u> seems to like.

Now, some of the famous people of the past in history that did snore. Two of them were George II and George IV. Also, Emperor Otho did according to the historian, Plutarch. President Theodore Roosevelt was reported to have snored very loudly at least once while he was recuperating in a hospital. And Lord Chesterfield snored. Also, the great Winston Churchill was a snorer of, "35 decibel(s)."

As one author puts it: "Snoring respects neither social nor economic boundaries. Numerous presidents of the United States are said to have been impressive snorers, including Washington, both Adamses, Lincoln, Taft, and Franklin Delano Roosevelt. And, although it sullies his image a bit, the famed British lady's man, Beau Brummell, was known as a prodigious snorer, as were Churchill and Mussolini." (Lipman, page 5).

Other important people such as Roman generals would snore also: "Even in the military, where all things male are celebrated, robust snoring is neither envied nor aspired to. The illustrious Roman statesman Marcus Cato withered one of his generals by declaring, 'His snore is louder than his battle cry.'" (Lipman, page 4).

And for the ladies that fantasize about "Prince Charming" type individuals, Beau Brummel, the ladies' man snored. Snoring in fact has probably broken lots of fantasizing throughout the thousands of years of man's history. In fact, it has been stated in one book on snoring, "...mostheavy snorers I have interviewed...I have found that the use of separate beds was not the exception, but the rule." (Mosley, page 13). Coming to the reality that humans need to overcome problems and then put on ideal traits of character that do not annoy their neighbor, can be a shock to some people. But to reality we all must come and then seek!

And could you imagine a "Prince Charming" snoring this much?: "...not...aroccasional snore here and there during the night. A researcher at the University of Florida, in Gainesville, monitored a group of habitual snorers and found that their average output was not less than 1,015 snores per individual per night." (Editors of <u>Prevention</u> Magazine Health Books, page 363). How would you like to have a "Prince Charming" like that? There are more qualities to look at than just good looks of a "Prince Charming". Is the person loving, caring, comforting, non--snoring, etc.

It just shows that <u>all of us</u> are **human**! So let's all lighten up on the subject at least a little, even though it is a sometimes very serious subject, and let us start to work on our causes of the problem to eliminate or lessen snoring. And please do not take your problem of snoring as if you are "less-than" other humans just because someone shames you for snoring. It seems every human snores sometime.

But the good news is that there is help and/or cures for nearly every human also!!! And that good character that brings the good life to all can come out of it all!

It is of interest to note here about the author, Dr. Boulware: "A man whose snoring had nearly ended his own marriage, Dr. Boulware asked for and received a $100,000 research grant from the National Institutes of Health to find a cure for snoring." (Lipman, page 13). I recommend Dr. Boulware's book as given in the Bibliography, as well as the book by Dr. Lipman, M.D. Other good writers on this subject of snoring are also recommended throughout this book.

Frequency of Snoring

And now back to the time sequence of the history of snoring. Back in 1972, John J. Burt, Ed.D., and Benjamin F. Miller, M.D. wrote: "Approximately one out of eight Americans, women as often as men, makes some kind of unmusical sound nightly. It may take the form of a grunt, hiss, snort, gurgle, or an assortment of noises, and it sometimes assumes a surprising intensity. To indicate the nuisance value of this problem, The United States Patent Office has on file patents for more than 300 snore-curbing devices." (Burt and Miller, page 290).

And, "In 1978 a team of medical researchers led by Elio Lugaresi, M.D., conducted a study of the inhabitants of San Marino, an independent republic of 20,000 people in northern Italy. From a questionnaire on snoring and sleep disturbances, Dr. Lugaresi determined that 20 percent of all people who responded snored regularly, that twice as many males as females admitted to snoring, and that snoring in men and women appeared to increase with age. Between the ages of 30 to 35, 20 percent of males and 5 percent of females snored regularly. From ages 60 to 65, however, 60 percent of the men reported snoring and so did 40 percent of the women." (Lipman, page 13).

And in another study that Dr. Lipman, M.D. tells his readers: "In a 1983 investigation done in Toronto on the prevalence of snoring, questionnaires were given to 254 consecutive patients attending a family practice clinic in the city and 25 consecutive patients in a clinic in a rural community in northern Ontario. Despite the environmental and geographic differences, the results in each group were so similar that they were not separated in the analysis. 86 percent of the women said their husband snored. 52 percent of the women said they were troubled by their husband's snoring. 57 percent of the men said their wife snored. 15 percent of the men said that they were troubled by their wife's snoring. The majority of snorers were male, outnumbering the females 9 to 1." (Lipman, pages 13 and 14).

Another fact in chronological order to the progress of snoring research comes from the writings of Jane Brody in her 1982 book (copyright date): "For all the people it afflicts, snoring has not attracted much research attention. There are fewer than 100 papers in the medical literature that discuss it at all, and only a handful reflect good research." (Brody, page 305).

Sleep Disorders Centers

"Not long ago, no one seemed to know (or care) much about sleep disorders. But new findings on apnea, which began in the 1960s, woke up the medical community to the importance of sleep research and sleep disorder medicine. In 1976 the Association of Sleep Disorders Centers (ASDC) was established, and sleep disorders centers started popping up all over the country...For a list of sleep laboratories around the country write to the Association of Sleep Disorders Centers, 604 Second Street S.W., Rochester, MN 55902." (Editors of **Prevention** Magazine Health Books, page 364).

And fortunately, these Sleep Disorders Centers and all the other preventions, helps, and cures are available today. There is virtually no need to worry about having a good night's sleep anymore if help is sought from a good health care Professional. This is true for the gentle snorer as well as the snorer with health problems such as with sleep apnea.

As one author puts the distinction between the gentle snorer and the more family-disturbing snorer: "Over 40 million Americans snore. For some, snoring is no more than an occasional and innocuous habit. But for countless wives, it represents an unending nightly disturbance that turns what Milton called the 'kindly dew of sleep' into a disruptive, nerve-racking experience. No doubt this is what philosopher/author Anthony Burgess had in mind when he wrote his famous epigram: 'Laugh and the world laughs with you; snore and you snore alone.'" (Lipman, page 2).

Fortunately, thanks to **modern** research and information, we now have many more preventions, helps, and cures which are discussed here in this exciting book! And we have much research done on good character development in building better relationships towards the goal of having good and wholesome unity for all!

CHAPTER 2: WHAT IS SNORING?

The term, "snore", probably started with the legendary herald in the Iliad, Stentor. Snoring has been called a "Stentorian roar." Stentor was the herald in mythology with the very loud voice with a combined sound of 50 regular men. Further, Homer, hundreds of years ago talked of this Stentor as "brazen-voice".

Definitions

And the <u>New College Edition of The American Heritage Dictionary of the English Language</u> defines "snore" as follows: <u>"To breathe through the nose and mouth while sleeping, making snorting noises caused by the vibration of the soft palate...English snoren,</u> to snort." (Morris, page 1223).

And it further defines "snort" as follows: "To exhale forcibly and noisily through the nostrils, as a horse...To inhale forcibly through the nose or mouth and so produce from the soft palate a vibratory snoring noise." (Morris, page 1223).

And, <u>Webster's New International Dictionary</u> defines snoring as "breathing during sleep with a rough, hoarse noise due to vibration of the uvula and soft palate." (Lipman, page 17).

Snoring is the unpleasant noise made by random movements in the mouth that cause vibrations when a person is usually sleeping. This is shown in the writing of Dr. Lipman, M.D.: "However, most ear, nose, and throat specialists subscribe to the definition that snoring is 'any resonant noise produced in the upper respiratory tract during sleep.' But the descriptions of that 'resonant noise' vary widely, from snorting, rasping, choking, and gasping, to rattling, sawing, rumbling, and hissing." (Lipman, page 17).

The World Book Encyclopedia tells us what snoring is also: "SNORING is a rough, broken sound made during sleep. Almost everyone snores occasionally, but men usually snore more often than women and children. Snoring usually takes place when a sleeper breathes through the mouth." (World Book, Inc., page 442, S-Sn, Volume 17).

And the question as to where the sounds of snoring originate can be found in a number of articles and books on snoring. For example, Dr. Lipman, M.D. says, "Snoring originates in those parts of your upper air passages called the collapsible part of the throat, or the collapsible airway. By collapsible, we mean that the soft tissues of this region have no rigid framework or support. They include the soft palate, uvula, tonsils, tissues around the tonsils (called tonsillar pillars), the base of the tongue, and the back and sidewalls of the throat." (Lipman, page 24).

John Burt, Ed.D., and Benjamin F. Miller, M.D. tell us what snoring is also: "Snoring is caused by vibrations in the soft palate and other soft structures of the throat when they come in contact with inflowing and outflowing air. The position of the tongue, enlarged tonsils or adenoids, a blocked nose, a bent or twisted nasal septum, and nasal polyps or growths can all be responsible." (Burt and Miller, page 290).

The Medical Doctor, Dr. Isadore Rosenfeld, puts it this way: "Why...don'twe snore during waking hours? After all, snoring is part of the breathing process, and all of us breathe twenty-four hours a day."

A further medical explanation of snoring follows: "Inspired air flows into the mouth and nose through the airways in the head and the pharynx on its way to the lungs. While we're awake, muscles in the area keep all these passages open, so the air rushes through them unimpeded. But when we sleep, those muscles relax, and the airway passages tend to collapse. Air now flowing through these constricted passages encounters resistance, requiring a greater inspiratory force. The resulting vibrations in the surrounding tissues constitute the snore. Its intensity, or loudness, depends on the degree of narrowing of the airways and on whether the tissues in the area are loose enough to 'rattle in the breeze.'" (Rosenfeld, page 73).

And another book written by Jane Brody an, "...award-winningand immensely popular 'Personal Health' (columnist)...of The New York Times since 1976: 'Snoring is the audible symptom of a blocked airway during sleep. The noise is caused by a vibration in the soft palate as the lungs pull hard to take in the diverted or weakened current of incoming air. The blockage may result from any number of circumstances, and these offer clues to alleviating the problem. Obesity, nasal deformities, and enlarged tonsils and adenoids may create structural obstacles to air. Nasal allergies, heavy smoking, gluttonous bedtime eating, and heavy consumption of alcohol and food can swell nasal passages and similarly block the free flow of air. Snoring is also more likely to occur among people who sleep on their backs; the tongue falls back toward the throat and partly closes the airway.'" (Brody, page 304).

One Medical Doctor at the University of Pittsburgh Medical School shows that even medical problems can be the cause of snoring of which one should seek proper Professional Medical care. He says that snoring is, "...vibrationsbrought about by more than a quivering of the faucial and velar tissues, but may be caused by anything which alters the normal contour of the nasopharyngeal passages, or swells the tissues and thus temporarily blocks part of the free air." And, "If snoring had the quality of a pleasant voice or musical tone, perhaps the majority of listeners would not be annoyed. A fundamental pitch forms the basis for the human voice, while an unrhythmic or non-periodic noise constitutes the fundamental snore. In sonorous breathing, the noise factor drowns out the resonant overtones coming from the vocal cavities and therefore is usually annoying." (Boulware, pages 35 and 50-51).

Conditions That Make a Snore

In general, five conditions must be met to make a snore: 1) The position of the tongue is back; that is, it is away from the front of the mouth and towards the throat. 2) The tongue must move into a position of being raised at its base. 3) The soft palate (also known as the velum) must be drawn back and drawn-up. 4) This soft palate and its little projection called the uvula that you can see if you look in the mirror (it looks like an appendix) must be loose so that it can vibrate freely. These here cannot be rigid. 5) Deep breathing in the amount of causing the chest to move enough to cause various amounts of air necessary for the snore. These are the five necessary ingredients that are needed so that the soft palate and back of the tongue are in just the right position to make the soft palate vibrate with its uvula due to the necessary amount of air in and out from the movement of the chest. These random mouth movements, making that all to familiar sound, are the "snore".

One author describes the workings of the uvula to produce the snore this way: "A long uvula may narrow the opening from the nose into the throat as it dangles in the airway. It acts as a flutter valve during relaxed breathing and contributes to the noise of snoring. An inflamed uvula usually caused from chronic snoring makes matters even worse." (Mosley, page 40).

And The World Book Encyclopedia gives this explanation as to the production of the snore: "Snoring takes place when a sleeper breathes through the mouth. Air rushing out through the mouth vibrates the soft palate, the soft tissue in the roof of the mouth near the throat. This vibration produces the sound. As the soft palate vibrates, the lips and other mouth tissue, cheeks, and nostrils also may vibrate. The rushing air dries the soft mouth tissues, causing them to vibrate faster. This makes the snoring louder." (World Book, Inc., page 442).

Levels of Snoring

Snoring can have different sounds to it depending upon which structural parts the air of the breath travels over the most. For example, if the air enters the throat in relation to the tongue base, which is what usually takes place when one sleeps on his/her back, then the resultant sound are a weakly amplified air draft that creates a noisy and raucous snore. But if there is the soft palate and inflamed uvula involvement, then the snore is minimal and very weak.

Thus, the reader can now see that there are various levels of snoring. And these levels have been described by physicians according to the state of health and other factors of the snorer: "To obtain a more precise frame of reference, physicians have developed an objective classification system for the degree of noise produced by snoring." (Lipman, page 18).

These are listed by Dr. Lipman, M.D. as follows: "**Mild**: Occasional snoring, usually while the sleeper is lying on his back and is overtired or has drunk too much alcohol or eaten too much food. **Moderate**:   Frequent snoring that occurs in all body positions. **Severe**: Very loud snoring that continues throughout the night in all body positions and can be heard from one or two rooms away. **Heroic**:   Extremely loud snoring that can be heard from three or four rooms away or throughout the entire house." (Lipman, pages 18 and 19).

CHAPTER 3: WHY SNORING? WHAT DOES IT MEAN? CAUSES

As early as 1906 in the <u>North American Review</u>, on October 5, 1906, an article was written that showed the part we all have in overcoming snoring. It showed that snoring means that a portion of our lives is out of control or unmanageable until we apply the helps and/or cures necessary to overcome the snoring. It shows that sometimes we just have to change our life-style.

Here it is: "...snoring...Excuse upon the grounds of unpreventability is absurd. If snoring was merely an obnoxious utterance of unconscious emotion, it might be woefully endured, but in fact it is a purely physical manifestation of the excessive indulgence in food and drink, or of ignorance of good form in recumbency. We may conclude generally that, 'early to bed, early to rise,' continues to produce the beneficial effects accorded by tradition to the habit, and that less turning of night into day would add materially to the sum of human happiness." (Boulware, page 24).

This is further emphasized by the great William Shakespeare, the English dramatist and poet, who wrote hundreds of years ago in <u>King Lear</u>, IV: "Our foster nurse of nature is repose." (Daintith, page 187).

So to get our lives back into control, we need to use the tools of modern health Professionals who know how to overcome snoring, and who know how to direct us to a better life-style, becoming our means to a happier and more productive life. We need to all adopt a precious life-style in order to avoid ever having an unhappy and painful life due to snoring.

For example, snoring can bring about this very painfully emotional and mental situation that no one would ever want to experience and can be avoided when snoring is prevented, helped, or corrected: "Dick's record of being fired from eighteen jobs in twenty years was the worst record of all the snorers I've interviewed, but poor job performance or loss of jobs is commonplace among heavy snorers. This darker side of snoring is due wholly to the snorer's daytime sleepiness. Individuals who suffer with daytime sleepiness are generally attacked when they are in the sitting position--they easily doze off into slumberland." (Mosley, page 21).

And James Mosley further quotes, by permission, the pamphlet of the American Sleep Disorders Association, showing that snoring had better be dealt with by a good health care Professional: "Extremely loud, habitual snoring is the first indication of a potentially life-threatening disorder, obstructive sleep apnea...snoring is no laughing matter! It means that the airway is not fully open...Perhaps one in ten adults snores and, for most, snoring has no serious medical consequences. However, for an estimated one in one hundred persons--typically, overweight, middle-aged men--extremely loud, habitual snoring is the first indication of a potentially life-threatening disorder, obstructive sleep apnea (apnea, a Greek word, means "Out of breath.") (Mosley, pages 22 and 23).

Then, James Mosley continues his own thoughts that show that good health care Professionals should be sought because, "People with this disorder don't breathe properly during sleep. As a result, they don't get enough oxygen, a lack that may contribute to excessive daytime sleepiness and trigger high blood pressure, heart failure, heart attack and stroke." (Mosley, page 23). More will be said about sleep apnea in the chapter 20 "Other facts about snoring and/or sleeping" located towards the end of this book.

Snoring is further an indication of possibly three categorically common causes according to Hinderer, an ear and throat specialist at the University of Pittsburgh Medical School 1) Medical conditions such as age, allergic related problems that bring inflammation to the nose, and endocrine gland hormonal problems. 2) Personal habits that are contributing to snoring such as lack of exercise, too much drinking, too much eating, and smoking. 3) Structural problems relating to the respiratory tract area.

The first of these is Medical conditions such as age, allergic related problems that bring inflammation to the nose, and the endocrine gland hormonal problems. Here Dr. Lipman, M.D. gives allergies as one of the "Common Nasal Causes of Snoring" in which he says, "About one in ten suffers from allergic reactions during his life. Most upper respiratory tract allergies result in swollen mucous membranes inside the nose and, consequently, obstructed nasal breathing; hence snoring." (Lipman, pages 33 and 34).

Receding Chin

The first two of these are discussed in greater detail throughout this book, but a structural problem that affects the respiratory tract area that needs to be mentioned is that of the receding chin, for which a good health care Professional should be sought: "Certain anatomical factors, such as a receding chin, can cause the tongue to protrude backward and aggravate the normal falling-back effect that already has occurred during sleep." (Lipman, page 28). Of course, with all the helps, preventions, and cures noted in this book, this too can be worked with to give even this snorer hope!

What Snoring Means: Consequences to the Body

And it is important to note what snoring means to the body's health as a consequence. "Snoring disturbs the patterns of the snorer. The blood is depleted of oxygen, so the heart must pump harder to circulate enough of the oxygen the body needs. Furthermore, heavy snorers tend to develop high blood pressure and show irregularities in their heart functions." (Mosley, page 43).

And this is again pointed out in Prevention's Giant Book of Health Facts: The Ultimate Reference for Personal Health, on page 309, R.I. Rodale's book edited by John Feltman, states, "Some research points to sleep disorders as a cause of hypertension. Sleep apnea (a breathing interruption), snoring, violent tossing and turning, panic attacks, and daytime fatigue are found in a disproportionately high percentage of people with high blood pressure."

And the Editors of Prevention Magazine put it this way: "But apnea doesn't have to be fatal to be harmful. It prevents restful sleep, which may cause 'disruptive and potentially dangerous physical and psychological side effects, such as personality change, sexual dysfunction, intellectual deterioration and hypertension,' says Thomas A. McCabe, M.D.,of Arlington, Virginia.

"And there seems to be a link between hypertension (high blood pressure) and the kind of chronic low-level oxygen deprivation that accompanies both snoring and apnea. 'People who snore every day, who snore loudly enough to make their spouses sleep in another room, put a tremendous amount of strain on their heart,' says Dr. Rice. 'It can create high blood pressure in the heart, and if it goes on long enough it might cause general high blood pressure.' This puts a double whammy on older men who may already be afflicted with circulatory problems. 'Snoring in most cases gets progressively worse with age,' Dr. Rice says, 'so that the strain on the person's heart and lungs gets worse just at the time when he doesn't want any extra stress.'" (Editors of Prevention Magazine Health Books, pages 363 and 365).

And Dr. Isadore Rosenfeld, Medical Doctor in his book on Modern Prevention: The New Medicine, shows the relationship of the simple snorer as well as the more complex snorer who has apnea to overall health: "Simple snoring and obstructive sleep apnea are really a spectrum, or continuum, in which men are afflicted twenty times more frequently than women. Such individuals tend to be stocky rather than tall and thin; they are likely to be overweight, to suffer from chronic lung disease, and, for some reason, complain of impotence. But perhaps the most important association is with high blood pressure." (Rosenfeld, page 74).

Then Dr. Rosenfeld continues to show the relationship of high blood pressure to sleep apnea. (See the chapter on sleep and other related snoring problems at the end of this book to learn more about sleep apnea and what it is). Dr. Rosenfeld says, "In a very recent study of some fifty men with hypertension, one-third were found to have sleep apnea--of which they were unaware. When the apnea was successfully treated, blood pressure dropped in most cases. On the basis of this and other related research, which suggest a 30 percent coexistence of the two conditions, it seems reasonable to look for the presence of sleep-related breathing disorders in all middle-aged or older men with high blood pressure." (Rosenfeld, page 74).

Types of snoring

Marcus H. Boulware, a speech pathologist and pioneer snore therapist, in his book, Snoring: New Answers to an Old Problem, on page 39 concludes that there are at least eleven types of snoring: 1) laryngeal. 2) nasal. 3) obesial (overweight as a cause). 4) Pseudo. 5) Neurotic. 6) Pathologic. 7) Physiologic. 8) Functional. 9) Lateral. 10) Supine. 11) Prone. A close look at these eleven types should lead the reader to a better understanding that Professional help is just what they, or any other person the reader would like to help overcome snoring, needs.

An example of what supine positions will do to a person that is prone to this problem of snoring is shown by John Burt, Ed.D., and Benjamin F. Miller, M.D.: "Most people snore only when lying on their backs, and an enforced change in position to prevent the tongue from falling back will prevent the snoring. An old remedy, dating back from the eighteenth century, stopped the snorer from sleeping on his back by sewing a hair brush to the back of his nightshirt." (Burt and Miller, page 290).

Then Marcus Boulware states: "Since many people snore only when lying on their back, they should train themselves to sleep on their side or stomach. For example, start by sleeping on a narrow, folding couch. It is miraculous how the subconscious mind prevents a sleeper from falling off the bed. When the lateral position is learned, the sleeper can move to a regular bed. When a snorer tells himself not to drift into relaxed sleep, at the same time he directs the brain to keep his mouth closed by repeating to himself, 'I will not snore tonight.' When this procedure is learned, then the sleeper can turn over the job to his subconscious mind which can gradually learn to control his snoring during relaxed sleep."

(Boulware, page 82).

Marcus H. Boulware further shows on pages 41-42 of his book that if the snorer has tightly closed his/her lips with their nose obstructed (for example, with a "stuffed-up" nose due to a cold or flu or allergy), then they may have a snore with a whistling sound. He states that when the nose has mucus congestion, hypertrophied horns, or polyps, and is thus narrowed so as not to allow healthy air flow through it, then 6,000 cycle per second violent sibilant tones may result associated with grave and irregular unsteady (tremulous) frequency. But if snoring comes from the lower part of the throat where the tongue has gone back into the throat making the throat tube diameter smaller, then a raucous and noisy, but weakly amplified air draft snore is created.

Point of Origin Gives Snoring Quality

It seems that it is the point of origin that determines the quality of the snore. This quality is like the different voices we all have, where the reader can tell who is speaking by the quality of voice the person has. For example, if the point of origin is the voice box, then the snore is of a raucous type but of weak volume which still might at times be strong enough to awaken someone out of their sleep and prevent someone from going back to sleep.

CHAPTER 4: PREVENTION OF SNORING (SCIENTIFIC)

In order to prevent anything, one must usually know the cause. This is because for every effect there is a cause. Therefore, the effect called snoring is brought about by certain causes. If we can prevent these causes from taking place forever, then we can eliminate the effect called snoring forever!!!

For example, if the cause is nasal congestion, "Just knowing the possible causes of nasal obstruction is of great value in determining whether or not you snore and where you might begin to look for factors that bring it on," says Dr. Lipman, M.D. (Lipman, page 33).

Some causes for snoring that may be familiar to the reader and has been shown to be a part of Kenneth Hinderer's (associate Professor of Otolaryngology at the University of Pittsburgh in 1974, approximately) approach to prevention and elimination of snoring are now to be mentioned. See if any of these seem to fit anyone's life-style, including your own, that you know to be a snorer. These are known as, "contributory personal habits."

Keep in mind that changes in the structure such as with inflammation or mucus of the upper respiratory area of a person leads to a change in air sounds called snoring. Also mentioned in some books and literature is the fact that it is the relaxation of certain muscles in the mouth and throat regions that contribute to the snoring. For example, Dr. Rosenfeld says, "While we're awake, muscles in the area keep all these passages open, so the air rushes through them unimpeded. But when we sleep, those muscles relax, and the airway passages tend to collapse...The resulting vibrations in the surrounding tissues constitute the snore." (Rosenfeld, page 73).

And with this in mind, Dr. Rosenfeld tells us, "You should avoid sleeping pills and/or alcohol at bedtime, since they increase the degree of muscular relaxation and so make the collapse of the airways more likely, thus increasing the obstruction to airflow." (Rosenfeld, pages 74-75).

And another author, Dr. Lipman, M.D., also gives another possible cause of the muscles relaxing in the mouth that result in the snore: "Each year, the coming of summer transforms many bedrooms into noisy torture chambers, according to modern snore lore. The reason: Scientists have shown that men snore louder and longer during the shorter nights of summer than they do in winter, and the fault lies with the sun. Longer days mean more chance to absorb ultraviolet rays from the sun, which produces more relaxation at bedtime. The more relaxed, the more vigorous the snoring." (Lipman, page 19).

And an encouragement to the reader is shown by John J. Burt, Ed.D. and Benjamin F. Miller, M.D., speaking about, "...common causes are...allergic conditions or colds which cause swelling of the mucous linings of the nose and induce mouth breathing, too much smoking, fatigue, overwork, and general poor health."

"Fortunately, many of these conditions can be corrected, either surgically or medically. For example, removal of enlarged tonsils and adenoids or of nasal polyps may give enormous relief. The use of certain drugs--antibiotics to reduce an infection, antihistaminics to shrink the nasal membranes, and steroid hormones--often clear up extreme nasal congestion." (Burt and Miller, page 290).

Another condition that needs to be mentioned as a cause of snoring is the person with, "An underactive thyroid or Down's syndrome...characterized by a large tongue which further blocks the upper airway during sleep." (Lipman, page 28). Here it would be wise for some people to check through a good health care Professional to determine whether they have an underactive thyroid that may be affecting their snoring. Probably not all low thyroids result in snoring unless it enlarges the tongue or other mouth area tissues or is associated with an inflammation of the mouth.

Smoking and snoring

The throat region (pharynx) of the heavy smoker can become changed. It may look "beefy", irritated, and red. This change in structure can be associated with snoring. It is called the, "smoker's throat." "From more than a dozen correspondents, I was informed that their snoring ceased when they gave up smoking." (Boulware, page 57). "And when specific factors, such as smoking are known to cause nasal congestion, avoidance should be tried for one month. With mucosal congestion, simple decongestive non-habit forming nasal drops may be the answer to correct the condition and stop the snoring." (Boulware, page 60).

And Dr. Lipman, M.D. says, "Smoking, though not a direct cause of snoring, contributes to it by causing the mucous membranes in the throat to swell and restrict the air passages." (Lipman, page 28). Dr. Lipman continues on page 34 of his book: "Tobacco, as we now know, irritates the mucous membranes and impairs the protective action of the nasal hairs, called cilia."

As John J. Burt, Ed.D., and Benjamin F. Miller, M.D., put it: "Other common causes are: allergic conditions or colds which cause swelling of the mucous linings of the nose and induce mouth breathing, too much smoking, fatigue, overwork, and general poor health." (Burt and Miller, page 290).

And unfortunately for those people who live in smoggy areas, the chances of snoring seem to increase, and it is worse to live in a smoggy area and smoke at the same time: "Allergies in the nasal passages are thought to be among the primary factors causing snoring, including industrial air pollution and cigarette smoking. One form of nasal allergy is 'allergic rhinitis.' This condition congests the nasal cavities and often leads to mouth breathing followed by snoring. All mouth breathers do not snore, but a great many of them do." (Boulware, page 61).

Eating abuse and snoring

The patient may eat mucous forming foods that cause the effect of postnasal discharge and/or edema (which is swelling of tissues) of the nose region. This can come from a heavy diet of carbohydrates. This in turn can cause the snore. "A Florida doctor described the case of a man who cured his snoring by a program of marked weight reduction; however, an old German medical dictionary stated that weight reduction induced snoring." (Boulware, page 57). And Dr. Rosenfeld, M.D. states, "Such simple measures as weight loss and regular exercise apparently do make a difference." (Rosenfeld, page 74).

And one book states, "The breathing blockage may also result from excess fatty tissues in obese people or from flabby muscles in the back of the mouth." (Brody, page 305).

This is further magnified by Dr. Lipman, M.D.: "Although the exact mechanisms by which obesity causes or aggravates snoring are unclear, we do know that the thick neck structures so frequently seen in overweight people tend to narrow the air passages. Moreover these individuals often have flabby tissues, with poor muscle tone, from lack of exercise...A long uvula and soft palate also reduce the size of a person's airway and increase the flutter-valve effect, which contributes to the sound of snoring." (Lipman, page 28).

"...Since obese and short-neck sleepers are prone to snoring, they should follow a weight-reducing regimen prescribed by a doctor. They should not be afraid to push themselves from the table." (Boulware, page 145).

And on this weight reduction, one book puts it this way: "Self-Care Remedies...Lose Weight. If you're overweight, shedding some pounds may be enough to solve the problem. For the average snorer, who is only slightly overweight, losing as little as 10 percent of body weight can make a dramatic difference, says Philip Smith, M.D., of the sleep disorders center of the Johns Hopkins University Medical School, in Baltimore." (Editors of Prevention Magazine Health Books, page 366).

Here in the above quotations, it is important to know that one needs good Professional health care since **how to** diet is very important. For example, loosing weight on a diet that builds mucous may produce a postnasal discharge. A good health care Professional's advice is therefore important and necessary. "The question of diet in the control of allergies, obesity, and overweight should be the province of the doctor in contradistinction to whatever influence folk cures and remedies may have." (Boulware, page 58).

Also, a diet that is high is salt may cause a retention of water or swelling in the nasal regions. One man wrote in Prevention Magazine, May of 1969, "About all heavy salt eaters I have known seem to have been snorers. My wife occasionally makes large kettles of soup which requires salt for the best flavor. But when she does, I notice a big increase of snoring in the family."

One author put it this way: "Overweight persons who have bulky neck tissues have a high probability of airway obstruction which produces snoring." (Mosley, page 42).

And another eating abuse is from eating ice cream that does not fit the person's health status: "Related to snoring are the constant wet nose and the commonly known postnasal drip. Both conditions stem from blood irritants. Blake F. Donaldson, in his book, Strong Medicine (Doubleday, 1962), reported: 'In order to add moisture necessary for oxygen interchange in the lungs to air that is breathed in, the nose needs to be reasonably well obstructed by turbinates--folds of membrane that give off moisture to the air going to the lungs...To supply the extra moisture to incoming air the nose needs a monstrous blood supply, so that the first place blood irritants running wild may be manifest is in the nose. Sneezing and snoring can be evidence of that. Many people will snore their heads off after eating ice cream for dessert.'" (Boulware, pages 62 and 63).

And discussing that condition called sleep apnea that can be associated with snoring, and is a problem more than snoring itself, Jane Brody says: "Sleep apnea affects the obese almost exclusively. Nine of every ten victims are male. Anyone with such snoring patterns who is excessively sleepy during the day (possibly dozing off while driving, while reading, or even while talking) or who has signs of memory loss or intellectual deficiencies would be wise to undergo a thorough medical examination and have his or her sleep patterns evaluated in a sleep laboratory...The apnea is often corrected by weight loss." (Brody, page 304).

Drinking abuse and snoring

The patient causes the throat to become irritated and swollen to various degrees which can cause variation in the quantity and quality of snoring. This is when the patient has an, "excessive and constant use of alcohol."

Dr. Lipman mentions alcohol this way: "Tranquilizers, antihistamines, or alcohol, taken in excess and prior to sleep, can aggravate snoring by deepening a person's sleep and causing even greater than normal relaxation of upper airway tissues." (Lipman, page 28).

Exercise abuse and snoring

Too much active exercise may induce excitement and tense muscles instead of producing muscular relaxation. But it is important here to note that proper exercise may help the snorer, unlike exercise abuse which may increase the snoring. Dr. Rosenfeld, M.D. puts it this way, "Such simple measures as weight loss and regular exercise apparently do make a difference." (Rosenfeld, page 74).

"Most of these conditions can be corrected and will respond to treatment. Poor habits of eating, drinking, and smoking must be eliminated, and the patient encouraged to substitute good personal health habits. In certain individual cases, a medical prescription may be found necessary; or a physician may find it necessary to instruct a snorer how to overcome his bad habits by exercising self-discipline." (Boulware, pages 56-57).

Dental Problems Associated with Snoring

One book takes a look at the possibility of dentures being a cause of snoring if they are improper in fit: "The breathing blockage may also result from excess fatty tissues in obese people or from flabby muscles in the back of the mouth--for example, when dentures fit improperly or are removed at night. Some find that sleeping with their dentures in place eliminates snoring, and weight loss usually does." (Brody, page 305).

Pregnancy and Snoring

51

Pregnancy should be a wonderful time in the life of all members of a family. When the woman is very healthy, it is my opinion that snoring will not occur with the pregnancy. But when there are toxins in the system that may be associated with congestion and/or allergies, the structures in the back of the mouth that flutter from congestion and/or allergies cause snoring.

Dr. Lipman, M.D. writes about pregnant women this way: "Similarly, a pregnant woman might become confused and embarrassed when she suddenly begins snoring. If she realizes that nasal congestion is a common occurrence in the early stages of pregnancy, and may be the reason she breathes in through her mouth, she will be more at ease." (Lipman, page 33).

Allergies and Snoring

Although the subject of allergies is mentioned throughout this book in relationship to snoring, a few extra facts on the subject may be helpful to the reader.

For example, in dealing with hay fever, Dr. Lipman, M.D. has this to say: "...hayfever might contribute to snoring without ever being spotted as the culprit. If the sufferer is lean and fit and is a non-drinker and/or a non-smoker, he might futilely resign himself to his snoring as some quirk of nature and never realize that it's due to his seasonal allergy." (Lipman, page 33).

And Dr. Lipman continues, "About one person in ten suffers from allergic reactions during his life. Seasonal allergies, such as hay fever, are caused by sensitivity to grass, tree, flower, and weed pollens that drift through the air at certain seasons of the year. Perennial allergies, to house dust or cat hair and the like, usually produce persistent nasal congestion accompanied by copious watery secretions and bouts of sneezing....Most upper respiratory tract allergies result in swollen mucous membranes inside the nose and, consequently, obstructed nasal breathing; hence snoring." (Lipman, page 34).

Medical Tests to Prevent or Detect Problems

In order to see whether one has a sleep disorder, tests may be made. These tests can help the person who snores to see whether they have a problem other than the snoring itself. As Dr. Hensel, M.D. puts it, "...they will provide valuable diagnostic information and may help your doctor to plan your treatment." (Hensel, page 226).

For example, the EEG, or electroencephalogram is, "...used to diagnose seizures, to investigate sleep disorders...The EEG is performed by placing electrodes on your scalp, then recording the tiny electrical impulses that are your brain waves...A specially trained EEG technician should perform the test, and a specialized neurologist should evaluate the results." (Hensel, pages 226-227). "'A clinic will give you a physical examination, and ask several hundred questions to find out your medical history, life-style, and psychological state,' says Rawlings. 'Then, if we suspect a serious sleep disorder, such as apnea, we'll conduct an overnight evaluation in the sleep lab. Different machines measure body functions such as brain waves, eye movement, breathing, oxygen saturation, heartbeat and leg movement. It is expensive. It might cost $500 to $1,500 for a full sleep evaluation. But we are also developing home monitors, which may be cheaper. I think that in the future, these will become widely available.'...For a list of sleep laboratories around the country write to the Association of Sleep Disorders Centers, 604 Second Street S.W., Rochester, MN 55902)." (Editors of Prevention Magazine Health Books, page 364).

And The World Book Encyclopedia (copyright 1983) has this to say about remedies for snoring; although, it should be kept in mind that this was written in 1983, we now have much better methods to choose from: "Many remedies have been tried to stop snoring. Bandages have been tied around the chin to the top of the sleeper's head so that the mouth would remain closed. A hundred years ago doctors removed the <u>uvula</u>, a tab of soft tissue hanging from the roof of the mouth near the throat. Attendants at an English hospital even tried dropping tiny soap pellets into a snorer's mouth whenever he made the sound. But doctors have never discovered a sure way to prevent snoring." (World Book, Inc., page 442).

CHAPTER 5: PREVENTION OF SNORING (COMPANIES, ETC.)

There are various companies and other people such as Nutritionists, Naturopathic Doctors, and others involved in alternative health care that deal with prevention of snoring. These companies and alternative health care Professionals have much to offer the reader. Again, it must be kept in mind that these companies and alternative health care Professionals are very important in helping anyone overcome or even prevent snoring; but a good health care Professional such as a Medical Doctor should also be consulted. And on the other hand, when consulting a Medical Doctor, it is good to have two or more opinions before one makes their final decision. And alternative health care Professional care can work nicely coupled with a wise Medical Doctor.

For example, Dr. Bernard Jensen, Nutritionist and a Doctor of Chiropractic has this to say about snoring: "Sometimes snoring hinders good sleeping. A good remedy is to place a small quantity of sesame seed oil or peanut oil in each nostril before retiring. This prevents drying out of the nose. Drying automatically opens the mouth, and snoring begins. It is claimed that this oil treatment is as effective as the sledge hammer or rolling-pin." (Jensen, page 55).

CHAPTER 6: PREVENTION OF SNORING (PEOPLE'S EXPERIENCES)

Different people have experienced different situations and have come to personal conclusions on how to prevent snoring. Some of these are familiar to different individuals. They may be familiar to some of you readers. I have found this true.

One of these is familiar to myself; the situation was different in that the people involved were different. It is written and experienced by Dr. Isadore Rosenfeld who writes the following: "...fromthe houseguest whose bedroom was next door to mine. I tossed and turned, but there was no way to escape the auditory assault. Apparently both our beds were similarly positioned with headboards against the dividing wall. Then a brilliant idea came to mind. I reversed position so that my feet steadied the wall. I hoped this would at least reduce the vibration. It didn't work." (Rosenfeld, page 71).

That did not work for him, nor did a similar situation work for me. In my case, I have been in hotels and motels where the person snoring very loud was disturbing my sleep. I tried to move my head in different positions and even place one of my ears on my arm with the other ear having a finger in it. None of this prevents the sound completely; although, this technique prevents some of the sound. From experiences like this one, I learned that true prevention comes by elimination of the cause of snoring which is explained in another chapter in this book and will be explained in this chapter also.

It can be frustrating to the individual to only be treating the effects and not the cause. These effects are the symptoms. I remember hoping and literally praying to fall asleep so I would not hear that ugly noise.

In fact, Dr. Rosenfeld continues his story: "What to do? I had no cotton with me, so I plugged my-ears with tissue paper. Totally ineffective. Then I did something I personally reserve only for the gravest of emergencies-I took a sleeping pill. (Remember I said earlier in this chapter it was alright to do so in an acute crisis. Boy, was this ever a crisis!). I waited for the merciful veil of sleep to descend, but every time it was about to do so, a staccato roar pierced it." (Rosenfeld, pages 71 and 72).

This might be familiar to some of you readers. If so, what did you do? Dr. Rosenfeld continues: "I did accomplish one thing that unforgettable night. You know how some people count sheep when they go to bed? After returning resignedly to my room, I actually tallied the number of snorts in an eight-hour period. Would you believe 926? That's right. Over an interval of roughly 480 minutes, 926 snorts--in singlets, couplets and short bursts. That works out to approximately two bursts per minute. In the morning, I never said a word about what had happened during the night. But when my patient invited me to stay the rest of the weekend, I suddenly remembered a very important appointment back home." (Rosenfeld, page 72).

I, too, had such an experience. My wife and I were trying to sleep at a hotel, but the noise of snoring roared into our room. I tried to ignore it, but my wife could not. Therefore, in the middle of the night, I had to go to the front of the hotel to get another room. The next room and our neighbors were both a delight, no snoring.

But once again, this is only treating the symptoms or effects of the cause. Some of the real causes of snoring according to the experts are overweight, smoking, allergies, eating abuse, and exercise abuse. This was discussed in an earlier chapter. Other causes are simply being too tired, in which case the recommendation to overcome the cause is just plain, "Early to bed and early to rise."

So, overcoming some of the causes is very important. And even not being tempted to do any of the causes is very important.

CHAPTER 7: HELP IN OVERCOMING SNORING (SCIENTIFIC)

There is much more research that has been accomplished by the time this book has first been written in late 1991 than there was in earlier years. This is because we today have much more knowledge and understanding thanks to greater technology and computers than in earlier years.

As Dr. Lipman, M.D. put it, "Until the early 1980s, however, there was little help for the snorer beyond fitting his partner with earplugs. As a physician, it was as frustrating for me to turn a patient away as it was for the patient to leave without getting relief. Around that time, reports of improved techniques in the diagnosis and treatment of snoring and related sleep induced breathing disorders began to appear in the medical literature." (Lipman, Preface, page viii).

Also, former knowledge has been added to or else eliminated due to findings that its clinical applications have not been as successful as hoped for, or better ways and means are developed. We can all be very thankful that new and more modern technology is always possible to help us all now and in the future to overcome or help in problems dealing with such subjects as snoring.

Antisnoring Devices

For example, on the subject of antisnoring devices, Marcus Boulware, on page 55, warns that if a patient has a nasal obstruction, chin straps and mouth dams, "could well endanger the health of individuals." He says that if a person buys them without the Medical care and observance, this could be harmful. He further notes that if the person has good nasal air passage, then the person may have the, "answer," if it is a functional snoring problem. Further, he states that these should be discarded after the person learns to control his snoring; or else, they become crutches and the snorer will not progress to a higher level of life in which he uses the method of self-control.

And a word of caution of why a person should work with a good health Professional in dealing with certain devices: "One who has studied snoring, Dr. Kenneth Hinderer, and ear, nose, and throat specialist at the University of Pittsburgh, points out that people normally breathe through their noses while sleeping, but if the nose doesn't bring in enough air, mouth breathing is used to supplement it. Snoring may result (though some people manage to snore with their mouths closed). He goes on to note that devices that attempt to eliminate snoring by keeping the mouth closed can interfere with an adequate oxygen supply to the body and brain." (Brody, page 305).

Tongue Retaining Device

James Mosley writes about mouth devices such as the orthodontic appliances that are, fitted in the mouth and some are structured to hold the jaw firmly in place or to bring the jaw forward during sleep. Some elevate the soft palate and others provide varying airway clearance. He talks about the TRD or tongue-retaining device in which a Dr. Samelson, "claims that more than 800 patients have been fitted with the TRD and the clinical success rate is over 80 percent." (Mosley, pages 65 and 66).

And on the Tongue Retaining Device (TRD), one book put it this way: "Similar to an athletic mouthguard, it forces you to breathe through your nose. In non-obese patients whose nasal passages are clear (sometimes this requires surgical repair of a deviated septum

60

or other blockage), the TRD is effective in 89 percent of the cases, says Charles F. Samelson, M D., of Rush-Presbyterian-St. Luke's Medical Center, in Chicago. The TRD is available only through sleep centers." (Editors of <u>Prevention</u> Magazine Health Books, page 365).

Here it is important to note that a dentist in Fremont, California, Dr. Alvarez, "is certified in the use of oral appliances to treat snoring...He started working with Dr. Samelson in 1985...His success rate using the TRD to treat snoring and sleep apnea has been over 80 percent..." (Mosley, page 65).

"There are over 120 dentists around the country who have been certified in the fitting of the new model TRD. For a current roster contact: R.Michael Alvarez, D.D.S., Medical-Dental Education Network, 38503 Botany Green, Freemont, CA 94536, (415) 793-3582." (Mosley, page 66).

Treatment of Allergies

Another help for snoring used by, "the physician," for snore provoking inflamed nasal conditions, is to, "...prescribe mild nose drops and oral antihistamines for relief from nasal mucosal congestion. This may eliminate snoring, but the patient should be told that this is only a temporary treatment. Treatment of the cause of desensitization to the specific antigen, or local treatment for sinus infection, is necessary to correct the cause of the mucosal congestion." (Boulware, page 59).

Inflamed nasal conditions can include allergies. The Medical Doctor can be consulted here: "Another cause of snoring which may be traceable to allergic rhinitis can appear seasonally or perennially. The seasonal type results from hay fever, pollinosis, and rose fever--with the additional symptoms of red eyes, itchy nose, and sneezing....any topical vasoconstrictor is effective, with preference for the aqueous solutions; epinephrine is effective in reducing nasal mucous membrane edema... Allergists sometimes recommend filters and air conditioners of all types to relieve hay fever sufferers and accompanying ocular symptoms. With the clearing of congestion in the nose, free breathing should eliminate the snoring." (Boulware, page 62).

And another book comments on allergies: "Nasal congestion may be relieved by eliminating allergens in the bedroom (dust, down pillows or quilts, non--foam mattresses), taking antihistamines or decongestants, stopping smoking, avoiding excessive consumption of food and alcohol in the evening, and reducing salt intake." (Brody, page 305).

And a comment about the position one takes at night is given by John Burt, Ed.D., and Benjamin F. Miller, M.D.: "Most people snore only when lying on their backs, and an enforced change in position to prevent the tongue from falling back will prevent the snoring. An old remedy, dating from the eighteenth century, stopped the snorer from sleeping on his back by sewing a hair brush to the back of his nightshirt." (Burt and Miller, page 290).

One author later quotes the pamphlet of the American Sleep Disorders Association showing the need to eat correctly and control one's weight in order to control sleep apnea: "Diet, if you are overweight. People with severe sleep apnea are almost always overweight. Even partial weight loss- 20 pounds by a 200-pound man who should weigh 165, for example- will improve breathing during sleep, make sleep more restful, and diminish daytime sleepiness." (Mosley, page 61).

"The American Academy of Otolaryngology pamphlet on snoring suggests for adults who are mild or occasional snorers to try the following self-help remedies:

1. Adopt an athletic lifestyle and exercise daily to develop good muscle tone and lose weight.

2. Avoid tranquilizers, sleeping pills, and antihistamines before bedtime.

3. Avoid alcoholic beverages within three hours of retiring.

4. Avoid getting overtired; establish regular sleeping patterns.

5. Sleep sideways rather than on the back.

6. Tilt entire bed with head upwards (place a brick under the bedposts at the bed head).

7. Allow the non-snorer to get to sleep first."

On commenting on number 5 above, Dr. Boulware, Ph.D., states: "The stertorous breather should train himself to do two things with the lateral sleeping postures: to breathe through the nose, and to sleep on his side. While experimenting with various sleeping postures, I found that 90 percent of the time I could sleep without snoring while lying on the left side, and probably 80 percent of the time on the right side. The lateral sleeping position seems to discourage mouth breathing, and this can be assured by placing the forearm under the chin to hold the mouth closed." (Boulware, page 101).

And one author gives a paragraph on what can be used to help overcome snoring, which are not cures but helps: "Finally, there are numerous tricks to maintain a snore-inhibiting sleeping position, such as stacking up pillows or a head rest so that the sleeper is more upright. Sleeping in a cervical collar (the type used to treat a neck sprain) will keep the chin elevated and often prevent snoring, according to one expert. Some have tried sewing

63

a marble or rubber ball into the back of the pajama top, which prompts a quick return to one's side. But avoid barricades that prevent the sleeper from turning over from side to side, since Dr. Hinderer's studies indicate that this may make matters worse." (Brody, page 306).

Muscle Training

And in discussing the subject of exercising the throat region muscles to help the person not to snore or perhaps cure snoring, Dr. Boulware, Ph.D. suggests the following: "Any muscle training which can keep the mouth closed has been considered one remedy for stertorous breathing. In carrying this idea further, I developed exercises to tone up the muscles of the soft palate. They are based upon the principle that the velum fluttering between two streams of inspired air produces snores. By using phonetic (speech) exercises to give tonus to the muscles which tense this organ, it can be concluded--at least theoretically--that snoring will cease. For instance, ah could be one of the exercises to tense the muscles of the soft palate, keep it closed, and prevent it from fluttering into snores." (Boulware, page 104).

And one book gives some other helps in overcoming snoring: **"Avoid Depressants.** Avoid central nervous system depressants such as tranquilizers, antihistamines, sleeping pills and alcohol within two hours of retiring. In one study, men who had one milliliter of 100-proof vodka per pound of body weight (for a 200-pound man, that's about two drinks) before going to bed had five times as many apneic episodes as they did when they retired sober, says A. Jay Block, M.D., of the University of Florida College of Medicine, in Gainesville." (Editors of Prevention Magazine Health Books, page 366).

And speaking about "**Drugs and medicines**" which are listed as one of the "**Common Nasal Causes of Snoring**", Dr. Lipman, M.D. makes some interesting comments of which the reader should always be under good Medical care while performing in dealing with drugs or medicines: "Aspirin, oral contraceptives, and estrogens--to name but a few drugs--can bring about endocrine changes that affect the nasal air passages...Decongestants...repeated use actually irritates the membranes and creates further nasal obstruction...A number of drugs used in the treatment of high blood pressure can also lead to chronic congestion and obstruction." (Lipman, pages 33-35).

And a book talks about the use of a cervical collar: "Wear a Cervical Collar. It's a device that's usually prescribed for people with sprained necks. Most snoring occurs when the sleeper lies on his or her back with the chin resting on the chest. That position narrows the windpipe. The collar keeps the chin up and the windpipe open." (Editors of Prevention Magazine Health Books, page 366).

CHAPTER 8: HELP IN OVERCOMING SNORING (COMPANIES, ETC.)

There are a number of companies and other non--scientific sources that can help the reader to overcome snoring. This is not to say that these are not based in science; but rather, that these helps are present for the reader to buy as presented by companies or others that do not have necessarily a health care Professional's license.

And the reader should note that these helps are just that, helps. That is, they are not necessarily preventions or cures. And they should still be showed to your health care Professional just in case your body cannot tolerate one of these devices or helps. For example, a special pillow used to help in overcoming snoring may cause a problem to a snorer that has a neck problem. In that case, a good health care Professional such as a Medical Doctor and/or a Chiropractor should be consulted **before** using the pillow.

And the reader should not loose sight of the fact that there are more than one kind of help in snoring. There are pillows, noise machines, etc. The reader can try one or more of these devices and/or helps. I personally have used a number of these and find them more effective when I can use more than one at a time. But I have further learned that preventive measures and cures are much more effective.

For example, I feel that I would rather learn how to go after the cause rather than treat the effect. This can be seen in the case of a person who is overweight or smokes or has an allergy. All of these have been shown in this book to be causes of snoring. If any of these causes are removed or overcome, then the snoring will stop permanently if these are the cause. (Sometimes there is more than one cause which is why it is wise to be under a good health care Professional's care).

To remove the cause is much better than to suffer with the effect. Would you rather live with a snorer using some kind of help like ear plugs or a noise machine, or would you rather only have to use the ear plugs or noise machine for a while knowing that the snorer will be cured soon? My desire is to see the cause removed so that I will not have to listen on an ongoing basis.

CHAPTER 9: HELP IN OVERCOMING SNORING (PEOPLE'S EXPERIENCES)

Dr. Isadore Rosenfeld, M.D. says this about people's household remedies: "There is no harm in trying these maneuvers; they may occasionally help." (Rosenfeld, page 75). This should be remembered when the reader reads this chapter; this is only a section on "help", not prevention nor cures.

Household Remedies

Dr. Isadore Rosenfeld, M.D. continues about household remedies used to help: "Scores of household remedies have been suggested over the years to control snoring, none of which really work." That is they may occasionally help, but they do not **cure** the condition. Good Professional health care should be sought for overcoming the snoring."

Dr. Rosenfeld continues: "I know patients who have tried all kinds of devices and contraptions varying from a neck collar to adhesive tape in order to keep their mouths closed. Since snoring is loudest when you are sleeping on your back, some desperate spouses have sewn little pockets on the back of their tormentor's pajamas in which they have inserted tennis balls or marbles to force them to sleep on their sides." (Rosenfeld, page 74).

But, people's experiences can be very helpful in dealing with snoring when one couples these with good Professional health care counsel. Experiences also show us that we are not alone in this world. We are not the only ones with the problem of snoring. And it gives us insight into possible ways that may also help us. The only caution here is that what works for some people may not work for others. This is why professional counsel is so important.

Good Attitude

James Mosley gave himself warm fuzzies emotionally and mentally in helping to overcome his chronic snoring problem. He says it this way: "I found out that it requires the same amount of energy and effort to form bad attitudes as it does good attitudes. I wrote some positive statements about every aspect of my life, and repeated those statements aloud numerous times each day. Four of my daily affirmations were, 'I believe I now get a good night's sleep. I do not snore. I sleep well. I feel good the next day.' I can now say that these affirmations and others have been fulfilled. I firmly believe that 'you are what you say all day long.'" (Mosley, page 62).

Folk Remedies

And Dr. Boulware, Ph.D. has given some folk remedies and non- folk remedies: "The following remedies have been suggested from many sources. If you snore, why not give them the 'acid test.' (Boulware, page 145).

"...The Japanese, according to an ancient legend, do not snore because they use a wooden pillow while sleeping. It is a block of wood 4 to 6 inches in height, and the person rests his head on it in such a manner that his head is tilted back and snoring cannot occur. (At least, that's the way I heard it. It is up to you now!). (Boulware, pages 145 and 146).

And on this idea, one book writes: "Self-Care Remedies...Prop Up the Head of Your Bed. Put a brick or two under the forward bedposts, Dr. Fairbanks suggests. This elevates the head and helps keep the airway open. Don't use extra pillows--they'll only kink the airway." (Editors of Prevention Magazine Health Books, page 366).

"...Charles W. Eliot, editor of the Harvard Classics, found it beneficial to go to sleep ahead of the snorer. This helps the non-snoring listener to get a head start in sleep. No less than a dozen people have recommended this first aid." (Boulware, page 146).

"...When sleep-inducing mechanisms are operating in the bedroom, they seem to discourage the snorer from being noisy. At the same time, they can put the non-snorer, to sleep...One such device...a Noise Box...did not cure his snoring, it simply made it more bearable to his wife...I have put myself to sleep by turning a portable television set off-station. The sizzling and peppering sounds lulled me to sleep in no time at all." (Boulware, page 146).

And one other book talks about the music box: "Self-Care Remedies...One is a music box, meant to be clamped onto the pajamas, that coos 'roll over, darling' when you lie on your back. Fortunately, there are some simpler approaches that doctors have found may be effective in some cases..." (Editors of Prevention Magazine Health Books, page 366).

"Autosuggestion is powerful if one has faith in it and perseverance. The snorer should say to himself: 'I will not snore tonight.' It ought to be repeated hundreds of times in order to be reinforced and stabilized." (Boulware, page 146)

"...A woman in Utah said that she used to roll over on her back while asleep, and, of course, she snored like a locomotive. To remedy the problem, she used two pillows and propped them against her back so that she couldn't roll over. She has been sleeping this way for the last four years, and there are no more snores." (Boulware, page 147).

And another book tells of the use of the "snore ball": "**Wear a 'Snore Ball.'** Since sleeping on your back increases the likelihood that you'll snore, one old-fashioned remedy is to sew a marble into a pocket on the back of your pajama to encourage sleeping on your side or stomach. Or make a bigger pocket and put in a tennis ball." (Editors of <u>Prevention</u> Magazine, page 366).

Then talking about the uses of honey in discussing **Folk Medicine** Dr. Boulware, Ph.D. knowing that there is an association between snoring and congestion in the nose writes: "Some of the other uses of honey include treatment for stuffy nose, nasal sinusitis, hay fever, and so on...the treatment of stuffy noses, post-nasal drip, and other nasal obstructions which may cause snoring. Treatment with honey caused stopped-up noses to open in three minutes and runny noses to dry up in five minutes. In addition, the treatment will also stop snoring in most cases. And chewing honeycomb will keep the nose dry--a very good prevention procedure which also stops snoring in numerous cases." (Boulware, pages 151 and 152).

And speaking on another **Folk Medicine** Dr. Boulware, Ph.D., gives this about cider vinegar: "...Sincea congested nose often causes an individual to snore, it is interesting to observe that wetness of the nose ceases with use of vinegar through the process of dehydration. An excess of mucus disappears and the proportion of moisture to the body becomes normal...Individuals with the problem of water nasal discharge were warned to omit foods made from wheat and replace them with rye and cornmeal foods. Patients were advised to eliminate citrus juices and fruits to clear up a postnasal drip." (Boulware, page 152).

CHAPTER 10: CURES IN OVERCOMING SNORING (SCIENTIFIC)

We are very blessed to be living in the 1990s since we have much more scientific studies about snoring than in the earlier years. For example, Marcus Boulware, a pioneer snore therapist describes the slow gathering of information on the subject this way: "Since 1955 only eight such (strictly medical treatment(s)) papers (dealing with scientific studies) have been published." (Boulware, page 49).

Marcus Boulware further states at the time of his book which was 1974, that some methods have proven ineffective; and he states that the doctor should be familiar with these, "which have consistently failed to cure snoring, or have been insufficiently tested," up to 1974.

These methods that he points out that have failed to cure snoring, or have been insufficiently tested are: "1. Amputation or excision of the uvula. 2. Injection of paraffin into the soft palate. 3. Injection of a sclerosing agent into the velum. 4. Prescription of snore prevention devices for use by patients with nasal obstructions." (Boulware, page 53).

On page 94, Dr. Boulware, Ph.D., mentions some of these prevention devices, in which he cautions their use with children: "...most of these devices are too bulky or painful for children to wear. Generally these devices restrain the sleeper from turning over on his back, such as wood cuffs and snore balls; mouth restrainers which curb mouth breathing, such as plastic gums or breathing dams; and neck extensors, made to prevent throat structures from rubbing against one another." (Boulware, page 94).

Surgery

He then explains on page 54 that he had his uvula removed as a possible cure for his

72

snoring, "but it was a failure." He says that this procedure has been discontinued for at least 100 years. Then he states, "Uvula resection may lead to disturbance of deglutition and speech." Deglutition is the ability to swallow, for example, one's food.

And Dr. Rosenfeld, M.D. adds the following: "An important caution: Most local surgical interventions used as a 'cure' for snoring--for instance, correcting deviated septums, and removing tonsils and adenoids--don't really have much impact on the problem. So think twice before you subject a loved one (to the extent you can still love anyone who does this to you night after night) to an operation." (Rosenfeld, page 75).

Dr. Rosenfeld then talks about snorers that are intense snorers: "However, if none of the approaches I have mentioned above succeed, and if you are dealing with a true 'mega-snorer,' the level of intervention may have to be raised." (Rosenfeld, page 75).

And another book talks about surgery also: "**Surgery**. UPP (uvulopalatopharyngoplasty) is the surgical treatment of choice for apnea, says Dr. Rawlings. Described as a 'facelift for the throat,' it calls for the surgical removal of the extra tissue that is blocking the airway. UPP was first meant for the treatment of sleep apnea, but turned out to be a remarkably effective treatment for plain old snoring." (Editors of <u>Prevention</u> Magazine Health Books, pages 365 and 366).

And with the care only of a good health care Professional, the following may be tried in our discussion of surgery: "Surgery may be needed to correct certain structural defects, such as deviated septum. But Dr. Hinderer suggests first trying to equalize the pressure in the nostrils by rolling up a tiny ball of tissue (from a piece about the size of a postage stamp) and placing it inside the pocket in the forward part of the tip of the nose. If the

73

pocket is bigger on one side than the other, he suggests a slightly larger ball of tissue on that side. This, Dr. Hinderer says, helps to open the nostrils and change the direction of the air current through the nose, so that the air will no longer cause a vibration of the soft palate, or snoring." (Brody, page 305).

Continuous Positive Airways Pressure

And then Dr. Rosenfeld brings out the use of the CPAP of which a qualified good health Professional can be sought. He says, "A relatively recent and effective technique for dealing with severe snoring and obstructive sleep apnea is referred to as CPAP--continuous positive airways pressure. This is a relatively simple and inexpensive treatment in which a small plastic mask is placed over the patient's nose. Room air, not oxygen, is delivered from a compressor at the bedside at a pressure slightly above normal...Synchronized with the patient's breathing, air flowing at such positive pressure keeps the airways from collapsing and hence stops snoring and sleep apnea. CPAP is the first route to follow. It often works." (Rosenfeld, page 75).

And on this CPAP use, one book puts it this way: "**Mask.** CPAP ("continuous positive airway pressure") solves the problem of airway blockage by feeding the sleeper a stream of pressurized air through a nose mask, from a bedside tank. 'These devices are still kind of cumbersome, but I have no doubt they'll get it down to a neat little space-age package in the next few years,' Dr. deBerry says. According to one University of Florida study, CPAP reduced the average number of snores per night from 1,000 to 23." (Editors of Prevention Magazine Health Books, page 365).

In fact, James L. Mosley in his book, Snore No More!, says about himself, a former

74

chronic snorer: "I have successfully used my CPAP system for more than three years. Shortly after I started using CPAP, I conducted my self-noise test. That tape was free of snoring sounds. This fully convinced me that CPAP works. I adapted easily to using my CPAP system and rarely sleep without it. I now feel great during the day without the daytime sleepiness I experienced before. My overall outlook on life has become much brighter." He continues, "I had found something that would stop my snoring...At the time I was using a Sleep Easy II N CPAP system, made by Respironics Inc...".(Mosley, page 71).

Then later James Mosley gives the address and phone number of Respironics Inc. on page 79 of his book:

Respironics, Inc.

1001 Murry Ridge Dr.

Murrysville, PA 15668

Phone Number: 1-(412)-733-0200 or 1-800-EASY USA

I had the pleasure of talking to them on the phone yesterday (November of 1991) in which Respironics told me about their program. I need to ask that all readers dealing with Respironics work through their Professional Medical Doctor. And, to remind you again that all readers should check with their Medical Doctor before doing **anything** found in this book.

And it should be encouraging to the reader what Dr. Barbara Gothe, at Veteran's Administration Hospital, says about the CPAP: "The success rate with my patients on Nasal CPAP is high, it's more than 80 percent...Careful patient evaluation, proper determination of the correct amount of air pressure required by the patient, along with patient compliance are all essential components in the high success rate with my patients." (Mosley, page 66).

Then Dr. Isadore Rosenfeld continues by telling his readers what to do if the CPAP does not work successfully. "If all else fails, and especially if the problem is one of sleep apnea, there is an operation that may help. This procedure, called UPP (which stands for uvulopalatopharyngoplasty), involves removing any excess tissue in the back of the throat that may contribute to the vibrations resulting from the constriction of the air passages. The UPP operation is no more complicated than a tonsillectomy." (Rosenfeld, page 75).

And as a last resort, Dr. Feldman, M.D. recommends the following: "Finally, in some cases when the sleep apnea is life-threatening, a tracheostomy may have to be performed. An incision is made into the windpipe, and the patient breathes through a tube inserted into that opening, thus bypassing the constructed airways higher up. This is really an emergency procedure of last resort and is never used just for snoring, no matter how bad. The tracheostomy is left in place as long as the circumstances leading to the sleep apnea persist. Frankly, if I had to live the rest of my life as I spent that one night in the Caribbean, I would recommend surgery--any surgery--without hesitation, even for severe snoring without apnea. But don't you let yourself get talked into it." (Rosenfeld, page 75).

Psychiatric

And no discussion on the cures of snoring would be complete without mentioning the psychiatric and psychotherapist: "For a patient with a snoring problem, psychiatric help may prove too costly...But if an individual's snoring is cured and family harmony is restored, it may be worth every penny expended. However, the average snorer will not require such treatment--probably one out of 100,000 snorers needs psychoanalysis to rid himself of sonorous breathing." (Boulware, page 78).

Then Marcus Boulware continues on page 82: "PSYCHOLOGICAL TREATMENT: Not every case of snoring has its origin in some neurosis or psychosis, and indeed such patients are rare. Since almost everyone has some kind of neurosis, a snorer with a neurosis may find it profitable to consult a clinical psychologist for treatment. Should a sleeper have only a mild case of functional snoring, he can experiment with the power of autosuggestion for curbing his abnormal breathing; if unable to understand and direct his own course of therapy, he should confer with a psychologist concerning autosuggestion and hypnosis." (Boulware, page 82).

Then Marcus Boulware later states how this autosuggestion has helped him: "I have used some of the principles of autosuggestion in seeking to rid myself of snoring. For instance, I learned what I call 'threshold sleeping,' that is keeping between the borderline of sleep and wakefulness during each cycle of sleep. This control was exercised consciously at first, while, at the same time, voluntarily using the jaw muscle to keep the mouth close. Then I turned the task over to the subconscious mind--I consciously kept myself half-awake and half-asleep until the behavior was learned. Hundreds of hours of practice were required in this psychological learning process. Although 'threshold sleeping' was not as relaxed as deep sleep, it did minimize the habit of stertorous breathing sufficiently enough to permit others in the household to sleep for longer periods." (Boulware, page 83).

And in order to give more hope to all readers in curing snoring, a further suggestion is given by Dr. Boulware, Ph.D.: "The habit of snoring must be eliminated and overcome by exercising will power while unconscious in sleep. In carrying out 'snore-riddance instruction,'

77

the snorer should engage another person to awaken him whenever he begins to snore. Then when wide awake, he must repeat the procedure for control of the throat muscles before he goes to sleep again. By persistence and repetition, the snoring habit is finally broken." (Boulware, page 105).

CHAPTER 11: CURES IN OVERCOMING SNORING (COMPANIES, ETC.)

These can be very exciting because they give hope to the reader that the condition of the person snoring will be overcome permanently. These cures are what I look forward to, as I am sure that most of you readers do also. They mean that the snoring will come to an end; that the snoring will not just be overcome by temporary techniques, but rather, eliminated. These eliminations can come in two types. One that makes the snorer completely quiet at night as long as the device or cure is still used, and the other that truly eliminates the problem.

The CPAP unit that has been mentioned already in this book is a good example. I contacted one such company that gave me permission to copy whatever they have sent me as I find need for my book. They were very helpful over the telephone, also. I want to thank them as their material will probably be most appreciated by most readers, if not all, that read this book. The company is Respironics, and I have already cited some of their writings elsewhere in this book.

CHAPTER 12: CURES IN OVERCOMING SNORING (PEOPLE'S EXPERIENCES)

When it comes to cures used by people to overcome snoring, a number of interesting techniques can be given. Some of these are very serious in the eyes of the person writing about it; and some are rather only interesting.

One of the most interesting cures that probably works very well but should not be tried for obvious reasons was written in a book where the author was being funny and not serious in this one example: "Too bad George didn't see this ad running in the newspapers of the day: **I Can Absolutely Cure Snoring** by a simple remedy that all physicians will unqualifiedly endorse. No medicine, no mechanical contrivances; just a simple rule, which followed, does away with even the most aggravated cases of snoring. Send $1 to_____. Understandably excited, many snorers quickly sent in their dollar and just as quickly received this printed response: **An Absolute Cure for Snoring   Don't Go to Sleep.**" (Lipman, page 11).

CHAPTER 13: TESTIMONIALS ON SNORING: IN MARRIAGE

Much can be said about the effects of snoring on a marriage. "Interviews with 100 habitual heavy snorers and their spouses revealed that 70 percent had experienced some sexual problems-generally the snorer is simply too tired most of the time-and 90 percent indicated they had experienced some marital difficulties due to their mates' snoring. The good news is that this darker

side of snoring can be corrected." (Mosley, page 13).

This can also be seen as true because some people do not snore in general. This does not mean that they have never snored in their lives, but it does mean that their mates have never heard them. And the good news is that all people with proper Professional health care have a good chance in the 1990s to reach the delightful state of no snoring in general. For example, Dr. Rosenfeld, M.D. tells of this situation in his own marriage: "...I was fortunate enough to marry a woman who among all her other virtues does not snore." (Rosenfeld, page 71).

Dr. Lipman, M.D. put the hoped for end result this way: "It is my hope that the information in this book will help many of you, among the millions of snorers, to obtain relief and bring your long-suffering partners out of the spare room and back into the bedroom." (Lipman, Preface, page ix). That statement is also a goal of this book.

Dr. Rosenfeld, M.D., continued to talk on the effect of snoring on family life by saying: "I have since thought many times about what it would be like to be married to or to live with someone who snored like that man behind my wall. Sharing a bedroom would naturally be impossible. Even separate rooms wouldn't work unless the house was big enough, or the walls adequately soundproofed. I then realized that a discussion of the prevention and/or management of snoring might be very much appreciated by millions of people who are exposed to the one in eight among us who are serious snorers." (Rosenfeld, pages 72-73).

The most important point to remember, in my opinion, is to examine the attitude and character of **both** the snorer and the one listening to the snoring. The situation of a husband or wife snoring and waking up or not allowing the mate to fall asleep, does not need to end in a marital argument. It depends upon the approach taken by **both** the husband and the wife. Good Professional counselling is in order if either the husband or the wife is dysfunctional. Speaking about a heavy snorer he met whom he called Dick, one author put it this way: "Dick found a way by seeking medical attention for his Snorer's Disease and physiological and spiritual counseling to get his marriage back on track." (Mosley, page 13).

For example, if a snoring husband is awakened by an angry wife, a functional husband will be considerate of her. He will lovingly discuss the situation with her. He will be comforting, compassionate, and consoling. He will seek good Professional care and counselling.

This can be illustrated by an example given by Marcus Boulware, a pioneer snore therapist. He gives the story of a "shamefaced" man who went to his nose and throat Medical Doctor for help because he was disturbing his wife. Dr. Morris Fishbein, a medical columnist wrote the story that goes as follows: The wife was so disturbed by the husband's snoring that she insisted on him going into a Medical Doctor for examination. The Medical Doctor found a deviated septum in the husband's nose, corrected it , and the snoring stopped."

This is a example of a solution seeking husband, a husband who will work on his attitude to cure the situation by removing the cause, instead of stubbornly conflicting about it. Instead, he worked on the cause, his septum in his nose that was not in its right position which caused a snoring noise that his wife could not tolerate. He said, "She is a musician and she wouldn't mind my snoring so much except that I keep getting off pitch." (Boulware, page 51).

And this husband is a good example of the advice offered by the author, James Mosley, who has researched for years the subject of snoring, in his book, Snore No More!, on page 10: "Whenever snoring becomes disruptive to the life of the snorer or to family members, medical advice should be sought." I agree! There is so much help that the Medical Doctor can give. And coupled with his help is alternative health care such as good Chiropractic care, and companies that offer special devices and/or products that can be used successfully with the guidance and direction of good health care Professionals. The Chiropractic care will be discussed more fully in the chapter on Testimonials: miscellaneous.

And amongst the letters that deal with snoring in marriage, Dr. Lipman prints four of these in his book. I feel his book would help the reader if he/she wants to be even further enlightened on the subject of snoring. It appears to have a different flow in dealing with the subject.

He talks about, "Perhaps the most celebrated letter about snoring in matrimony came not from a woman but from a man. In April 1915, George Little of Pittsburgh, Pennsylvania, wrote to the <u>Ladies' Home Journal</u> asking readers for advice on how to stop his disruptive habit. Readers' replies poured in from all over the country with recommendations, information, and sympathy. So numerous were the responses that the <u>Journal</u> started a column that ran for a year, entitled 'How Can George Stop Snoring?' Eventually, the unending flood of letters from thousands of anxious readers forced the editors of the <u>Journal</u> to cry, 'Enough! If Mr. Little hasn't enough 'cures' by this time, the <u>Journal</u> fears he is hopeless!'" (Lipman, page 11).

One said: "I never used to snore until my hair began to fall out, and the balder I got the louder I snored...Finally my wife...brought from town one day a slumber cap, which I have worn ever since--at night, of course--and I have ceased to snore. You see, my hair was so thin that I caught cold every night, and stuffing up, would snore." (Lipman, page 10).

Another said: "Do you realize that Indians never snore? I have slept many a night in their tepees and never a sound. The secret of it is that Indian children are always taught to sleep with their mouth closed so as to prevent throat troubles. Here is a hint for mothers if we are to prevent another generation of snorers." (Lipman, page 10).

One respondent to my questionnaire, Karen Fritz, stated "Neither my husband nor I snore under normal circumstances. Sometimes, if he has a cold, he'll snore a little, but no major log-sawing. He says that occasionally, I snore when I lie on my back." Another wife, Gena Zerlan, comments that her husband's snoring "keeps me awake, tremendously irritates me in the night; I want to kick him out of bed." Gena's advice to help overcome snoring is "poke him, poke him, poke him!!!!!!!!!"

CHAPTER 14: TESTIMONIALS ON SNORING: ROOM-MATES

The pain associated with being a chronic snorer, especially a heavy snorer, is demonstrated by an author who has finally controlled his snoring. (You can order his book that is listed in the Bibliography if you desire. His book may help many of you.) But before his snoring was controlled, he relates his deep feelings: "The ridiculing that Dick faced because of his loud snoring is an experience that I have been confronted with many times. I soon began to avoid activities that required overnight stays away from home. I had become very sensitive about my snoring. I wouldn't share a room overnight with a non-family member, camping trips and retreats were a no-no for me--I just simply refused to go." And he continues, "I preferred self-confinement in my own bedroom rather than be subjected to ridicule and embarrassment because of my snoring." (Mosley, pages 17 and 18).

CHAPTER 15: TESTIMONIALS ON SNORING: BROTHERS/SISTERS

Snoring amongst siblings, brothers and sisters of a family, can be a problem in families. Stress can be the result, and often bad attitudes can result from the stress that builds in the brother or the sister. One respondent to my questionnaire wrote, "A younger brother of mine is a world-class snorer! We could hear it all over the house!!." It is important that the parents teach their children how to live in harmony with one another through the use of warm fuzzies.

Fortunately, some children, even if they have a snoring problem or not, have their own bedrooms and do not bother anyone. Dr. Rosenfeld, M.D. in his book tells it this way about his own experience: "I'd never had any great personal or professional interest in the problem of snoring. As a child, I was always lucky enough to have my own bedroom." (Rosenfeld, page 70).

It is important to note here the causes of snoring in children that need to be overcome to solve the physical problem. A good health care Professional should be consulted. For example, one author points out a physical problem that needs to be overcome since it can cause snoring. He states, "Excessive bulkiness of tissues in the throat, such as large tonsils and/or adenoids commonly cause snoring in children." (Mosley, page 42).

CHAPTER 16: TESTIMONIALS ON SNORING: PARENT/CHILD

Before beginning this section on testimonials on snoring as it relates to the relationship of the parent to the child, it is important to see what can be done for a child.

Dr. Marcus Boulware, whose "research for SNORING was conducted, in part, under the auspices of a Carnegie Foundation grant, " has this to say about children as related to snoring that parents can heed: "COPING WITH SNORING CHILDREN: Since infants and young children are unable to carry out muscular tonus exercise, and as antisnoring devices are too bulky for them, they must necessarily accept the treatment administered by pediatricians and dependable parents. In addition to the efforts of the physician, the parent or the nurse can be most helpful in reducing stertorous breathing through the following techniques: "Change the sleeping positions. Whenever the child turns over on his back, the child can be shifted to the lateral or prone position, since children who are mouth breathers snore readily if they are sleeping on their backs."

"...thereis an old saying that snoring will stop if a person is rolled over on one side. Fox and Kessel, physician and dentist respectively, stated there is more truth in this statement than we realize. They remarked that this has been observed in people with nasal allergies as is often the case with infants and children. If one is turned on his side, the opposite nostril will become open because the blood gravitates to the side on which the person is lying. This permits sufficient air to pass through the nose causing the mouth to close, and snoring is thereby eliminated."

"The child should be dressed comfortably for bed, but not overdressed because he will become overheated and develop colds that clog the air passages, causing nasal snoring." (Boulware, pages 93 and 94). Here it should be noted that proper ventilation is important in all four seasons in order to avoid stuffy noses. Avoid drafts in the winter, and if it is warm enough in the spring and summer, get plenty of fresh air. Pollen in the spring and summer may cause allergies that tend to produce snoring. Some authors I have read tell of getting good air filters. Dr. Boulware comments on a room that is too cold in the winter, and dust-laden in the summer: "Either may cause respiratory ailments which create conditions in the nose upon which snoring seems to thrive." (Boulware, page 94).

And Dr. Boulware, Ph.D. comments on allergies in children by telling his readers that they should be helped by the Medical Doctor. Here it is important to read the chapters in my book on alternative health care Professions that can be used in conjunction with the Medical Doctor. "If the child has symptoms of nasal allergies, take him to a doctor. An allergic condition indicates that the child is sensitive to certain foods, pollens, and perhaps certain liquids. If the condition is not promptly treated, the lining of the upper respiratory tracts become swollen and may lead to snoring. The family doctor will usually refer the child to a specialist trained in treatment of allergies." (Boulware, page 95).

And Jane Brody, an, "...award-winning and immensely popular 'Personal Health' (columnist for)...The New York Times since 1976..,"writes the following to consider: "Snoring is common among children under the age of ten, usually because of enlarged tonsils and adenoids or nasal allergies. It becomes less common during adolescence and young adulthood, only to increase again after the age of thirty." (Brody, pages 304 and 305; and front cover).

And very important to remember when dealing with children that snore as shown by Dr. Boulware, Ph.D. is, "Give love and understanding. Scolding a child for snoring is cruel, because he cannot control the condition. He does not have the knowledge to bring relief, and therefore parents must do this for him. Seek to discover the cause, demonstrate understanding, and give the required help." (Boulware, page 95).

CHAPTER 17: TESTIMONIALS ON SNORING: MISCELLANEOUS

There are numerous people that I have talked to that complain that snoring by themselves as well as others can affect their health. For example, if a person keeps waking himself/herself up by their own snoring, then less sleep is obtained. This can lead to being more tired the next day. Some people have told me that they can remember waking themselves up from snoring; they can remember hearing themselves at the very last moment snoring before they awaken. I have had that personal experience, also. I can remember hearing a sound that awakens me out of my sleep. Others have told me similar stories. In responding to the question of how do you feel about your own snoring, one person pondered, "I wonder if I do; I've never thought about it before."

And for me, I usually feel more tired that next morning. My eyes feel more sleepy, and I do not have a feeling of well-being. Fortunately, I have learned how to overcome this problem of waking myself up. I do this by following as many of the prevention methods of snoring found in this book.

While I am on the subject of what snoring seems to do to me, I would like to mention other symptoms that I have noticed on myself when I awaken at night due to my own loud noise. Being a Chiropractor, I am very interested in the musculoskeletal system, and I have felt my muscles upon awakening. Each time I have awakened I have noticed very tight muscles in the shoulder region and the neck region. When I massage these tight muscles for about five minutes, I never wake myself up again due to my snoring. My theory is that these tight muscles are associated with my snoring.

Chiropractic Care

Here I would like to mention that Chiropractic care is probably a good method, along with other good Professional care, in helping the person suffering with the problem of snoring. The reasons for this are probably many. For example, Chiropractic helps to reestablish the government or nerve supply back to throat, uvular, and muscular regions.

The Chiropractic adjustments of the spine help to bring the nerve supply back more fully to the areas that are lacking good government control of the nervous system. When it goes to the uptight muscles of the shoulders and neck, these muscles have a tendency to relax; this in turn helps a person to sleep better and more properly.

The Chiropractic adjustments of the spine further help to increase the nerve supply to the uvula and throat, making these areas healthier; and thus less susceptible to inflammation which has been said to be involved with snoring. This nerve supply further can help to bring more health to the cells of these regions so that they would have more power to clean away the mucous that would be present in mucous problems. Earlier references were made to the fact that mucous has been felt to be a contributing factor in the cause of snoring.

And the Chiropractic adjustments probably can help in snoring since they work with the major influencing system of the body: the nervous system. The nervous system is known to balance the body's functions. If the problem of a particular snorer is a functional one in which one or more of his organs are contributing to his snoring, then the Chiropractic adjustment may help.

I can still remember Dr. Cleveland of the Cleveland Chiropractic College in Los Angeles, California telling us to memorize the functioning of the nervous system due to its extreme importance in the over-all picture of health. He told us to memorize what is found in Gray's Anatomy, the 28th edition, on page 4. I still have it hopefully memorized perfectly as follows: "The function of the nervous system is to control and coordinate all the other organs and systems of the body, and to relate the individual to his environment. Therefore, any incoordination of **any** organ or system of the body may be helped. And if this incoordination is associated with snoring, then it follows that the reestablishment of the organ and system coordination may help the snorer."

CHAPTER 18: HUMOROUS SITUATIONS ABOUT SNORING

Although snoring is nothing usually to laugh about, some situations may be humorous **after** enough time has passed or after the person has been helped or cured of their problem. I used the word, "humorous" which is applied to a situation that no longer can be used against anyone but rather has a lesson to be learned within the story. Some people would rather use the word "funny"which is sometimes interchangeable with "humorous"; although, my experience in dealing with some sensitive people has lead me to avoid certain words like "funny". Please forgive me if you are a sensitive person to the word, "funny"as I am using it as if it means humorous.

The snorer usually does not realize that his snoring bothers people so much as he/she is asleep at the time; but their closest neighbors usually let them know, and it is not "funny" at that time. Usually in denial, the snorer cannot understand the seriousness of his effect on others.

Dr. Isadore Rosenfeld, M.D., puts it this way: "Can you name the one disorder in medicine that is characterized by the following? (1) The patient is totally unaware of the condition, denies that he has it and usually suffers no ill effects from it. (2) Those around him are perfectly miserable. (3) When convinced that he has a problem, the afflicted individual treats it as a joke, even though the impact on others may be devastating. Those characteristics identify the snorer." (Rosenfeld, page 70).

John Burt, Ed.D, and Benjamin Miller, M.D. put it this way: "Everybody jokes about snoring, but the various unpleasant noises made by 21 million snorers can be seriously disturbing to their unhappy listeners: Laugh and the world laughs with you. Snore and you sleep alone." (Burt and Miller, page 290).

And another book written by Jane Brody, has it written this way: "The bedroom is filled with snorts and chortles. A woman is perched, lamp in hand, ready to strike the somnolent source of the distressing sounds--her husband. This and similar scenes are common in comedies and in cartoons...Though often a subject of derision and humor, sonorous breathing during sleep, better known as snoring, is really no laughing matter. It's certainly no joke to those who have to listen to it and sometimes not to the creator of the grunts, rumbles, whistles, rasps, and hisses. In addition to its sleep-disrupting effects on spouses, roommates, and neighbors, snoring particularly the persistent, loud kind, can be a signal of a serious health problem." (Brody, page 303).

She also gives a quotation of a doctor that making jokes can discourage more research: "'Treating snoring as a joke discourages research and perpetuates our ignorance,' says Dr. Charles Pollak of the sleep clinic at the Montefiore Medical Center in the Bronx, New York."

Joking can sometimes do that. I have seen joking literally stop a good conversation, a conversation from which we could have learned from! We must know to whom we are telling our jokes. If the joke offends anyone, then it was not worth giving. Some jokes are only cold pricklies instead of warm fuzzies! The reader can understand this better by reading the chapter in this book on Warm Fuzzies.

Also, the reader or the one(s) that the reader has to listen to, if either of these snore, do not find snoring jokes too funny if they are in a lot of pain or are shame-based. I need

94

to emphasize that the reader be very careful not to use jokes to any person who is sensitive to the issue of snoring.

This is because, if they are shame-based, then the reader might hook their shame and loose a friend. Or else, the reader might get a negative response because the snorer might feel put down or feel less-than. But once a snorer has overcome his/her snoring, then it usually is safe, but still not always if the person is still shame-based.

Please know the person's present status if he/she is still a snorer or not; and then check for their sensitivity level first before telling any funny story. It is not a joke to people that are sensitive. Do not tell a funny story to someone that will be hurt by it! Quoting the pamphlet released by the American Sleep Disorders Association, James Mosley writes in his book, "If you snore loudly and often, you may be used to middle-of-the-night elbow thrusts and lots of bad jokes. But snoring is no laughing matter! It means that the airway is not fully open."

So let's all be sensitive enough to others feelings and thoughts as we find out <u>where they are at</u> in relationship to this sensitive issue! Some people are serious and highly emotional about the subject of snoring; let's only give them warm fuzzies that **fit** them in a **positive** way.

At this point it would be wise for the reader to read the chapter on Warm Fuzzies at the end of this book. This will give the reader ways to never hurt anyone that causes offense or disunity; but rather, it will show how to give warm fuzzies that will repair hurt relationships and build unity.

The rest of this chapter will cover what some other books or magazines or newspapers have written on the subject by their various authors. I hope you all enjoy every word, none is meant to be offensive in any way. Now sit back and relax, and perhaps laugh a bit!!!

Snoring Champions

One author wrote about snoring champions! How would you like to be the world's snoring champion? People could praise you for it instead of shaming you! Well in 1944, Harry Christy took over Idaho's snoring championship. He replaced the "too jerky" snoring of former champion W.H. Gilman of Twin Falls who held the title for seventeen years! (Boulware, page 22).

And how about this for championship snoring competition?: "The true snoring champion of the world is Melvin Switzer, according to the Guinness Book of World Records. Using recording equipment provided by the local Noise Abatement Society, mighty Mel outblasted his competitors during the early morning hours in a contest held at Hever Castle in Kent, England, on June 28, 1984. He proudly took first place with a snore score of 87.5 decibels--the equivalent of a motorcycle revving up at close quarters. (Note: Switzer's wife is deaf in one ear.)" (Lipman, page 6).

"It is of interest to note that 100 decibels is found with 'deafening' thunder and gunfire." (Mosley, page 7).

And another funny championship snorer contest is described by Dr. Lipman, M.D. in his book as follows: "Some of the truly outrageous snorers managed to capitalize on their vice. David Bishop, reputed to be the champion snorer of the great state of Arizona, was challenged by Texan Steve Hawkins to a Snore-Down. The bet was $10,000. The two men checked into adjoining rooms at a local hotel to do their stuff for the judges (the town undertaker and a magistrate), who stood outside the bedroom doors to evaluate the thunder." (Lipman, page 6).

Probably some of you readers know of some people who are champion snorers! The good news is that most every champion is replaced in the snoring field of champions when help and cures are put into **action**! Hopefully someday there will never ever be anyone else who will ever qualify for such an awful title ever again! Let's all work to bring that day into reality!

And this loud snoring is stated again this way: "'The loudest snore recorded so far has been 80 decibels,' says Dale Rice, M.D. of the University of Southern California, in Los Angeles. 'That's about the equivalent of a jackhammer ten feet away. Some have been the equivalent of a 747 taking off or the sound of a diesel bus at close range.'" (Editors of Prevention Magazine Health Books, page 362).

That would definitely not be humorous if anyone had to sleep next to this person. Fortunately, most snoring problems can be helped or cured. This person would probably be helped with good Professional care also; so do not be discouraged if a loved one or other person you know snores in a way that you feel is like this snoring champion!

Animals that snore!

Another funny situation, except while it is happening to someone, is when an animal snores. In the Introduction to this book I told of the story of my own dog, Kookie Burns, that snored. Other stories can be just as funny or more so.

And we need to keep in mind to be selective to whom we are telling funny stories about animals. Some people are going through problems with human snorers and their animals only increase the snoring problem. So be careful to whom you tell any funny story: "In our urban areas, sleeping humans often listen to noises at night as do their watchdogs. A number of different kinds of environmental sounds are listened to by men and women lying awake with insomnia, or in the anticipation of snoring from a companion. Some people can tolerate all kinds of loud, man-made industrial and traffic noises more easily than they can snoring--perhaps they dislike the snoring of animals as much as they do that of humans." (Boulware, page 163).

Marcus Boulware talks about animals that snore: "I concluded that nearly all domesticated, carnival and circus, marine and zoo animals snore at least occasionally. More specifically, they were elephants, camels, cows, sheep, cats, dogs, lions, horses and mules, chimpanzees, leopards, tigers, gorillas, zebras, oxen, elands, and buffaloes." (Boulware, page 157).

"Yes, cats snore...about midafternoon he generally stretched himself before the cozy fire, purred and made a snoring noise--though weak in volume...It appears that their air passages do not generate sufficient pressure for loud snoring. At least a dozen of my acquaintances have recalled that their childhood cat pets snored." (Boulware, pages 158 and 159).

And on the subject of dogs, one may want to choose their dogs as pets carefully. For example, "Long and slender-nosed dogs like collies have small anterior respiratory outlets and rarely breathe stertorously; and, if so, it is not loud enough to keep anybody from sleeping. But certain breeds of dogs...are given to snoring. Usually they have blunt faces, stenotic nares, elongated soft palates...dogs like the Pekingese, boxers, pugs, Boston terriers, and certain bulldogs." (Boulware, page 159).

And this is shown again by Jane Brody: "Animals, especially such blunt-faced dogs as boxers and Boston terriers, also snore." (Brody, page 305).

And what to do if your dog snores?: "If small domestic animals snore because of nasal infections or obstructions, the veterinarian treats them in a manner similar to that of human beings. Most owners of pets carry them to the veterinary hospital for treatment with amazing regularity at the first sign of illness." (Boulware, page 159).

And here is a funny story about a __?___. If I told you about this animal, it would ruin the funny story. See if you can pick out the animal before you have read the whole story: "The news media reported the story of a vicar who launched into his sermon one Sunday morning in Haydock, England. Suddenly snoring began...The parishioners all looked attentive, but the snoring grew louder. A feather drifted down from the rafts and the vicar relaxed, because it was Ossie, the owl, sleeping in the roof. 'Ossie's snoring sound is uncannily like a human being,' explained the church warden, George Petts. 'The vicar's face was a treat to watch the first time it happened.'" (Boulware, page 160).

And on the subject of horses and mules, see if you know of anybody who can snore in both positions that a horse can! If you know of anyone who can snore in both positions, please let me know!: "Some veterinarians have observed snoring among horses and mules. Horses can sleep standing up, but they may lie down in their own stables. It would appear that horses can sleep and snore standing up or lying down." (Boulware, page 160).

CHAPTER 19: WHAT PEOPLE THINK ABOUT THEIR OWN SNORING

Whether we are young or old, we each have our own opinions about our own individual snoring. Some people completely deny that they ever even once have snored. Other people tell me that they know that they snore because their snoring wakes them up sometimes.

But the saddest situations to me are found when someone shames themselves for snoring. This usually is not healthy shaming but rather toxic shaming in which the person belittles himself/herself for something that they cannot prevent--it is not always their fault! This is true also for the elderly as well as the young!

The elder person need not put a burden of shame on himself/herself just because they snore. Sometimes with age and inheritance factors and how the person has styled their life results in a change of muscle tone of the mouth region that can bring on snoring. Dr. Lipman, M.D. writes it this way: "Muscle tone in the tissues of the throat also slackens with age. (Just think of the sagging skin under an older person's chin.) As our upper airway tissues become more floppy and less resilient with age, even in our waking state, it isn't surprising that snoring increases significantly as people get older." (Lipman, page 28).

Let's see what one book writes: "You can stop losing sleep over your sleeping problems. Persistent sleep disorders that had been accepted as normal consequences of aging are now being researched and diagnosed in the many sleep clinics throughout the nation...People should no longer accept the 'common view of the average older person as someone who sits in front of a television set, on a park bench, or at a church gathering and falls asleep,' says Dr. Carskadon. 'Daytime sleepiness in older persons may be caused by too little sleep at night due to circadian rhythm disturbance, adverse effects of medication, or reduction of activity. Physiological sleep tendency may not necessarily be greater in the elderly than in younger adults." (Editors of Prevention Magazine, page 367).

There it is! Do not ever be too hard on yourself! But do find out the cause for your snoring and/or sleep disorder by working through a competent good health care Professional. In the above paragraph, for example, it may be that you need to get proper exercise, or have your Medical Doctor reevaluate your medicine, or just to be taught a pattern of sleep to reestablish your circadian rhythm. So if you are wrestling to stop snoring or to get to sleep, it may not be you as a person, but rather a change in your life-style may make a major change in your snoring or sleeping problem.

CHAPTER 20: OTHER FACTS ABOUT SNORING AND/OR SLEEPING

There are many other facts about snoring of which some will now presently be discussed here. Also, sleeping needs to be discussed relative to snoring in order for this book to be more complete.

The seriousness of sleep disorders is evident as shown by The Wall Street Journal's report on July 7, 1988: "Sleeping problems in the workplace--whether the result of irregular shifts or medical disorders--are costing companies an estimated $70 billion annually in lost productivity, huge medical bills, and avoidable industrial accidents. Sleep disorders, of course, are particularly frightening in areas affecting public safety. Researchers say that as more is learned about the economic toll of sleep disorders, companies will find they cannot afford to continue ignoring the problem. Megabucks are involved, and sometimes, lives." (Lipman, page 54).

Rapid Eye Movement Sleep

There is a special state of sleep called REM sleep or rapid eye movement sleep that appears to be the state in which the snorer snores. Dr. Lipman, M.D. points this out in his book: "During sleep, the degree of muscle relaxation increases with the depth of sleep, and the more relaxed the tissues, the greater the likelihood of vibration and the sounds of snoring. As we have seen, maximum muscle relaxation occurs during REM sleep--especially in the neck muscles. Most snoring occurs, therefore, during this period of sleep." (Lipman, page 26).

Dr. Lipman, M.D. has this further to say about REM sleep: "This phase is distinguished from other sleep stages by a dramatic decrease in muscle tone. The skeletal muscles of the neck, arms, and legs are essentially paralyzed. Breathing becomes irregular, the heart rate increases, and the eyes display rapid, darting movements. The soft tissues of the upper airway, including the tongue, soft palate, and uvula, are completely relaxed." (Lipman, page 22).

Sleep Apnea

But it should be kept in mind that snoring of and by itself may not indicate that the person is ill, according to some of the articles and books I have read. It is put this way by the Medical Doctor, Dr. Rosenfeld: "Snoring usually has no ill effects on the perpetrator. For example, my fellow guest in the Caribbean looked--maddeningly--great the following morning. Occasionally, however, respiratory pathways are so narrowed or constricted that the amount of air passing through them is very much reduced. This results in a condition called obstructive sleep apnea." (Rosenfeld, page 73).

And Jane Brody shows that simple snoring is not as bad as sleep apnea: "Most of the time snoring is intermittent and innocuous, except for its disrupting effects on the sleep of others. But some people snore all night, indicating a possible shortage of oxygen for a significant portion of a person's life. In turn, recent studies suggest, this may lead to daytime fatigue and eventually may precipitate high blood pressure and other disorders of the cardiovascular and nervous systems." (Brody, page 304).

She then continues, "In a few cases heavy snoring is a sign of a potentially life-threatening problem: sleep apnea, in which breathing stops for seconds or even minutes at a time and finally resumes with raucous snorting and tossing about. The pattern may be repeated hundreds of times all night long. The resulting chronic oxygen shortage may lead to abnormal heart rhythms, high blood pressure, and heart strain." (Brody, page 304).

It is hoped that at this point the reader can see the need to prevent, help, or cure the snoring, especially the heavy snoring and the sleep apnea type of snoring. If good health care Professionals are not found, health conditions can worsen. Snoring of all types is no laughing matter. But the good news is that there are many preventions, helps, and cures as can be found throughout this book!

Then Dr. Rosenfeld goes on to describe obstructive sleep apnea which only some snorers have, not all snorers: "An individual with this problem breathes in a characteristic cyclical fashion; first there is the familiar rhythmic snoring, followed abruptly by total cessation of breathing. The resistance in the airways is so great at this point that no air moves through them. The chest, however, continues to heave as if the person were still breathing, but he is not. The silence may last anywhere from a few seconds to as long as two minutes. During this time, since the lungs are not receiving air, the blood is deprived of oxygen, and so are the tissues throughout the body, including the heart and the brain." (Rosenfeld, page 73).

This of course can bring on undesirable health related problems. Dr. Rosenfeld continues, "When the oxygen concentration in the blood drops below a certain level, sleep lightens and respiratory centers in the brain stimulate the breathing mechanisms vigorously, so that air once more moves through the constricted passages. The period of respiratory 'arrest,' or apnea, ends with a particularly loud snort, followed by a succession of other 'bursts,' after which the cycle repeats itself--snore, silence, snort, paroxysms of snorts, and silence. The recurring drop in oxygenation has health consequences that include hypertension, behavioral alterations the next day and even sudden death during the night." (Rosenfeld, pages 73 and 74).

And Dr. Rosenfeld next tells of the consequences of how the individual feels the next day: "At the end of each cycle of apnea, the individual actually awakens, although he later has no recollection of having done so. Since this happens every few minutes throughout the night, the person with obstructive apnea is not only chronically oxygen-deprived, he also has a sleep deficit. He therefore tries to catch up during the daytime hours--sometimes involuntarily; literally falling asleep while conversing or even standing. This is called the Pickwickian syndrome, after the fat boy in Dickens' Pickwick Papers, where the description of this daytime somnolence was so classic!" (Rosenfeld, page 74).

From the books and literature I have read on the subject of sleep apnea, where the sleeping person stops breathing for short periods of time, there appears to also be much written. This sleep apnea, which has already been described, can be associated with snoring in which the snoring person will stop breathing at times. The results from this problem can be stressful physically, emotionally, and mentally to the snorer as well as to those around him or her.

The seriousness of this state of snoring, or some might say that sleep apnea is only associated with snoring since not everyone has sleep apnea even if they snore, is shown in the following statements: "Snoring can be more than just annoying. It can sometimes be the first symptom or the earliest stage of a serious respiratory disorder called sleep apnea, in which the sleeper stops breathing for ten seconds or more in episodes that occur seven or more times an hour. Apnea, which occurs in roughly 30 percent of heavy snorers, can be fatal, but in most cases a vigilant section of the brain has the presence of mind to change gears at the last moment and jolt the body into a lighter phase of sleep. The sleeper half-awakes, gulps in fresh air and saves his own life.

"But apnea doesn't have to be fatal to be harmful. It prevents restful sleep, which may cause 'disruptive and potentially dangerous physical and psychological side effects, such as personality change, sexual dysfunction, intellectual deterioration and hypertension,' says Thomas A. McCabe, M.D., of Arlington, Virginia." (Editors of Prevention Magazine Health Books, page 363).

Dr. Hensel, M.D. puts it this way: "If your partner snores at night, but is sleepy during the day, he or she may have 'sleep apnea.' This condition is caused either by a problem in the central nervous system or by a subtle and partial blockage in the back of the throat. It results in periods of time when less than adequate oxygen reaches the brain. As a result, the person is tired the next day, despite an apparently restful night.

"There are treatments for the disorder, which most often affects obese people and those with high blood pressure, but diagnosis can only be achieved if the condition is suspected and tested for. The test is performed to check for sleep apnea or to evaluate daytime sleepiness. It may also be used to evaluate the possibility of narcolepsy, a nervous system disorder that causes sudden, unexplained periods of loss of consciousness during the day. This test is not routine; it is complex and expensive and should only be done on appropriate people. Because it is safe, accurate, and non-invasive, however, it may be undertaken on those who are suspected of having sleep apnea or some other sleeping disorder. It is especially indicated for people who have all of the risk factors for sleep apnea: snoring, high blood pressure, obesity, and complaints of daytime sleepiness." (Hensel, pages 227-228).

One such writing on this aspect of snoring is found in a pamphlet written by the American Sleep Disorders Association and quoted by James Mosley in his book: "A particular pattern of snoring interrupted by pauses, then gasps, reveals that the sleeper intermittently stops breathing. Some people do not breathe at all for three quarters of their sleep time. "Such vastly disturbed nights produce profound day-time sleepiness that often disrupts work and personal life. People with sleep apnea fall asleep at inappropriate times, at work or behind the wheel of a car, for example. Recent studies show they have two to five times as many automobile accidents as the general population."

"People with sleep apnea may have trouble concentrating and become unusually forgetful and they may seem uncharacteristically irritable, anxious or depressed. These problems may appear suddenly or emerge over many years. The person may not notice them himself or may minimize their severity. Often family members, employers, or co-workers first recognize a pattern of changes in mood or behavior and prompt a visit to the doctor." (Mosley, page 23).

Another book put it this way: "The most common symptoms of sleep apnea are snoring and excessive daytime sleepiness, says Bernard deBerry, M.D., a Laguna Hills, California sleep specialist. Sometimes this chronic tiredness gets to the point where sufferers actually fall asleep on the job or while driving to work. Other common symptoms include: morning headaches, sexual impotence, personality changes, memory lapses, chronic depression and snoring that's remarkable because of its loud strangling sound (this, of course, is reported by family members)...If you suspect you have apnea, visit a sleep clinic, advises Rawlings." (Editors of <u>Prevention</u> Magazine Health Books, page 365).

And Jane Brody has this to say about sleep apnea associated with snoring: "The apnea is often corrected by weight loss. Sometimes surgical relief of a blockage in the nose or upper throat is helpful. Other cases may be helped by antidepressant drugs or nasal tubes, but some victims require a tracheotomy (a surgically created breathing hole cut through the windpipe) to eliminate the risk of fatal complications." (Brody, page 304).

The good news is that people with snoring and sleep apnea as a combination can be helped. After quoting the American Sleep Disorders Association, James Mosley is so encouraging to all people that have this problem or know of friends or loved ones suffering from it. He tells of a person named Dick who had such a terrible problem with sleep apnea and snoring and how this problem was overcome: "Dick was diagnosed as having severe (life-threatening) obstructive sleep apnea, but the good news is that Dick's non-surgical treatment stops his snoring, and eliminates his excessive daytime sleepiness. He has been on the same job for over two years now and has been promoted to a supervisory position." (Mosley, page 23).

In dealing with sleep apnea, The American Sleep Disorders Association gives treatments that may help: these include oxygen supplementation, medication, surgery, and tracheostomy.

The American Sleep Disorders Association says this about oxygen as stated in James Mosley's book, <u>Snore No More:</u> "Supplemental oxygen, administered during sleep, may help people whose blood oxygen levels fall significantly during apneas. These may include people with both obstructive and/or central apnea." (Mosley, page 62).

The American Sleep Disorders Association says this about medication: "The drug protriptyline (Vivactil) seems to benefit those with relatively mild obstructive sleep apnea. It also diminishes the level of snoring. It is believed to work by stimulating muscles around the throat, keeping the upper airway from collapsing. Unfortunately, it has a number of unpleasant side effects, including dry mouth, constipation, and urinary retention." (Mosley, page 62).

The American Sleep Disorders Association says this about surgery: "Surgery may be able to correct physical abnormalities that compromise breathing during sleep. These include enlarged tonsils or adenoids (far more common in children than adults), nasal polyps or other growths, a deviated nasal septum, and malformations of the jaw or upper palate. Using a technique known as the uvulo-palato-pharyngoplasty (UPP), a surgeon removes excess tissue at the back of the throat that may be a factor in blocking the airway during sleep. Studies show that the UPP benefits about half of those who undergo it...A few patients report troublesome post-operative effects." (Mosley, page 63).

CHAPTER 21: WARM FUZZIES

Warm fuzzies are the ways of life that mend and bond or unify our relationships. It is our responsibility to give **all** people around us warm fuzzies if we ever want relationships of love, joy, peace, goodness, gentleness, and self-control.

Love, because love is the outgoing expression which a warm fuzzie brings to the person to whom we give it to.

Joy, because happiness to the fullest is achieved when warm fuzzies keep coming, uninterrupted by the opposite of warm fuzzies which is cold pricklies. I feel special and warm inside when my wife or children or anyone else gives me warm fuzzies. This is especially true when I have done nothing to deserve them; or contrary, I was not in a good attitude and they gave me a warm fuzzie regardless of my attitude. The latter is an example of unconditional love which brings the highest kind of happiness and joy.

Peace, because when someone gives a warm fuzzie to any of us, we are given something special and fitting to us. This brings no resistance usually, and therefore only brings peace. When someone gives to me something I like, I am grateful and something inside wants to be more peaceful towards that person. And a feeling to have unity and bonding develops. This feeling can further develop into thoughts and action if the person and I continue to give each other warm fuzzies. Cold pricklies would have a tendency to offend or break any bonds of unity that are already present; and therefore, I try to avoid them.

There will never be unity and harmony of all humans on the earth as long as cold pricklies exit. Cold pricklies include such ugly activities and attitudes as lying, killing,

110

stealing, getting at the expense of others, spreading diseases, etc.

For example, an ugly cold prickly used by a woman who harmed a boyfriend just because he snored is as follows; and this kind of attitude and action should be forever removed from the face of the earth: "It's hardly surprising that snoring provokes such marital discord. 'We know of a woman in Texas who actually shot her boyfriend because he snored so loudly,' says David N.F. Fairbanks, M.D., an otolaryngologist at George Washington University in Washington, D.C." (Editors of Prevention Magazine Health Books, page 363).

Goodness, because warm fuzzies help to build relationships. Something good is something that builds. Like many of you readers, I want to see all people united someday in perfect harmony. To build such a great society, warm fuzzies are an absolute necessity. And these warm fuzzies must come from a source that understands equity and equality of people in a righteous way!

Gentleness, because warm fuzzies make the receiver of them want to maintain a gentle approach in order not to upset the blessing of the warm fuzzie. I have enjoyed warm fuzzies so much that I have tried not to upset the situation of the person giving them to me. I have learned, after 44 years of life, that I can spoil a warm fuzzie if I do not handle the situation carefully by giving back warm fuzzie attitudes back to the warm fuzzie giver. This requires gentleness. Therefore, another fruit of giving warm fuzzies is gentleness.

Self-control, because warm fuzzies are so precious. I therefore control myself so I do not loose the graciousness of the giver. Sometimes, my feelings and/or thoughts might not be appreciative of the warm fuzzie. In that case, the effect of the warm fuzzie on my life is not to the full; therefore, I have learned to enjoy to the fullest the warm fuzzie and its giver by connecting or giving my full attention through self-control. This self-control is the discipline I use in which I gain control of which thoughts and feelings I choose to have in order to maintain the precious situation of a warm fuzzie.

It needs to be shown at this point how this works when a situation of snoring comes about in one's life. But first, I desire to give to the reader an example of how warm fuzzies can work in their lives by a subject that seems to help in snoring situations. I wrote this article for the <u>Women's News</u>, for the December of 1991 issue. Keep in mind, while you read it, that massages will relax the snorer so that they seem not to snore as much from my experience. Here is the article:

ADD WARM FUZZIES TO YOUR LIFE-STYLE!

"Add warm fuzzies to your life-style! You'll be delighted that you did! They can warm up nearly **any** relationship! And after you have practiced them enough and have made them part of your character, the benefits are wonderful! They can bring more love, joy, and peace into your life! They are necessary in order to have the kinds of **healthy** relationships we all desire.

Warm fuzzies are the general ways of a life-style that need to be used forever. They are the ways we all want to be treated by others **forever!** Amongst a long list, they are the ways of giving, sharing, helping, comforting, giving compassion, and consoling. They come in all areas of a person's life-style: physical, mental, emotional, and spiritual.

Let's take an example of how to use these warm fuzzies in our lives. The example I want to use is probably one that you all desire to have done to you. It is that delightful feeling we all experience when we are **massaged**! And we all know that the experience is great only when the qualities of many warm fuzzies are used. The more warm fuzzies used the warmer and fuzzier is the massage.

I have seen in my twenty-two years of experience in giving over 100,000 massages, the benefits to people personally and in their relationships through good warm fuzzy massages. These warm fuzzy massages that are now given in my Advanced Massage Therapy office in Fort Collins, Colorado, have helped hurt relationships and have helped "good" relationships get better. By the use of the same warm fuzzies in your families, you too may experience these wonderful benefits. (Always check with your city and state to see if you can massage in your families by law. And check with your Medical Doctor to see if there are any contraindications.)

The first thing to know is that warm fuzzies must be as its name says, warm and fuzzy. So the room must be warm and comfortable, <u>not</u> a bumpy couch to work on in a cold uncomfortable environment. It might be nice to add some warm relaxing music, if the person so desires.

Which leads us to the second thing to know: always make your conversation personalized. This is a very important warm fuzzie. I have seen clients in my office that have enjoyed their massages because any conversation was about them. Sometimes they did not want to talk at all.

It is important to know the mood that the person being massaged is in. I have used the warm fuzzies of comfort and compassion in my massages, which builds a health bond between us. This can be used effectively at home to fulfill your overall mission of having

113

a unified and happy family.

For example, when I see any of my family members looking stressed, at the appropriate time I ask if they would like a massage. The massage starts out gently rubbing their backs until the muscles relax. This removes the effects of the stress they were under. This work on the person physically usually leads to giving to the person emotionally and mentally, and sometimes spiritually. This works wonderfully to open up the lines of communication with a mate or any of your children.

And at that time of open communications is a great time to bond or build more unity in the family. It is a time that "hurt feelings" or just building a better emotional bond can be achieved. And it is very important to remember the other warm fuzzies at this time. The more warm fuzzies used at a given moment, the higher the delightfulness or ecstasy in a family: the kind that we all dreamed and hoped for before we got married.

For example, a teenage daughter or son may be walking around the house in a depressed mood. This also applies to other people, too, such as a mate. After talking in comforting, compassionate, and consoling words to them, ask if they want a nice massage. Sometimes the asking of the massage has to come first before the warm fuzzy words. Once the muscles are relaxed, the family member is usually quicker to open up about the stress that is bothering him/her. Here I have learned to **never** use cold prickly words, but rather only helpful, comforting warm fuzzies.

In my Advanced Massage Therapy office, just like at home, I practice these very important principles or warm fuzzies. We all need to practice these because they then become a part of us. They become our character. This leads to confidence that we can help others in nearly any situation; because we see that we have the strength of character to do the warm fuzzies that lead to peace. And since that is our goal, to have and make peace in our own lives and in the lives of others, in a good healthy way, we learn to have a <u>heart</u> to love warm fuzzies forever."

And one more thing before we discuss warm fuzzies in relationship to snoring. We need to discuss how to overcome stress in our life and help overcome it in the life of the snorer. This is important since physical, mental, emotional, or spiritual stress appears to affect snoring. The following is an article I had published in the <u>Women's News</u>, the November of 1991 issue:

ATTACK STRESS ATTACKS!

Most stresses and their effects can be attacked leaving us in a goodly amount of mental and emotional serenity! This can be accomplished using a time tested method used by hundreds, if not thousands of people.

The method for attacking stress is through the use of setting boundaries which define and develop the self, and recovery or the elimination of old bad habits that block self development.

The method for attacking the effects of stress is by overcoming the symptoms such as tight muscles which can cause a person to be uptight, and emotionally and mentally nervous. I will come back to this important issue later.

Fortunately, there are solutions for overcoming the stress itself as well as the resultant symptoms. Of highest importance is setting of boundaries. Boundaries define and allow us to be involved in the creation process of ourselves as individuals. Think about it! You can make yourself the kind of person you want to be by choosing the qualities you want to be you, and then not allowing anyone or anything to stop its development. This is known as an attitude or positioning of your mind that you take towards people and things around you. When we practice these attitudes daily, we develop character which is what we are known to be.

To accomplish this, make a list of all the qualities that you want to be. Carry this list on paper and review and add to it throughout your lifetime. This is your forever list of things you want to become. These should be qualities of character that will result in leadership and the ability to get along with others on a forever basis. Leadership here is to lead people through modeling the example of life that leads to the character that produces serenity inside oneself.

The list can include such general qualities that all of us need in order to get along with one another such as love, trust, loyalty, forgiveness, and giving. Beyond these is a need for personal qualities such as personality traits that must be developed and nurtured subject to the general qualities of life. These can include such traits as creativity in a specialized field, exactingness, love to travel, sports likes and dislikes, food likes and dislikes, etc. Personal preferences as boundaries will bring serenity emotionally and mentally when followed since it is these that you yourself have chosen and desire.

One example of this attack on an invading stress could be where both you and your mate like to play tennis. Before you leave the house to go play, someone calls you on the phone and asks you to come over for lunch. You have been wanting to get together with this person for a long time. The resulting tension from this stress is mental and emotional conflict of which event to do. If you have the boundary of prioritizing, for example, then you can attack or overcome this stress by knowing that family usually comes before friends. This gives peace or serenity of mind.

Further, I have seen the results on the muscles and the spine for about twenty-two years now when people have chosen the way of peace verses the way of conflict. The muscles of the body seem to relax in the person with boundaries that help in bonding relationships. This results in the muscles pulling gently on the bones of the spine in such a way as to help maintain the bones of the spine in alignment. The lack of boundaries, for example in the above illustration if the person would have gone out with their friend instead of their mate, would only bring hurt feelings and mental and emotional pain. This in turn seems to make the person uptight which tightens the muscles nearly anywhere in the body, pulling bones out of their proper positions with possible resultant pain. Unfortunately, if this takes place in the spinal regions, nerve or governmental supply to the organs of the body will be decreased resulting in symptoms that bring more suffering to the individual.

I have personally treated hundreds and possibly thousands of people that have told me why they felt they had tight muscles in their body. I have learned that I can help to adjust their spines and release the tension on their muscles to help remove the effects of stress; but only the person can change themselves in order to attack the stress attack by the development of good character."

I have talked to some people who have read this article and have started to practice it. Also, people who I have told this to in the past have also noted a greater peace and serenity in their lives and have noted less complaints about their snoring. Personally, I have noticed that the building of good healthy boundaries in my life, and seeing this also in my wife, Pina, has helped us give each other more warm fuzzies than ever before; and both of us sleep more relaxed with snoring, even on stressful days, down to a minimum.

At this point it should be reemphasized that nearly everyone snores at some time in their lives. But the good news is that if we can get our life-styles under self-control (temperance); then even the times when stresses do attack our lives, we know how to bring the effects of stress to a minimum. This is important to note since, as has been shown in other chapters of this book, stress in the form of physical, emotional, mental, or spiritual can be associated with the causes of snoring. These causes include overweight, smoking, food abuse, drinking abuse, exercise abuse, etc. As the other chapters show, these lead to swelling and excessive relaxation of the throat and mouth tissues which leads to snoring. An example of this is allergies from eating abuses.

CONCLUDING REMARKS

Thus, I hope that this book will bring many happy days into your lives and the lives of your friends and loved ones! Many people have asked me to write this book as soon as possible since they suffer personally from the problem or else know of someone who has snoring as a problem. I tell them to buy other books or go to the library. And that my book will soon be available that will hopefully coordinate much of the other information. So, I hope that you readers have enjoyed this book and will look forward to my next edition, bringing you more and updated information on snoring.   In this book, I have aimed to bring to you a crystal clear knowledge, understanding, and wisdom; balanced with the approach of love, compassion, comfort, and consolation that all of us humans so deeply need. Hopefully, my book has provided the reader with a method to grow mentally, emotionally, and spiritually throughout the pain of overcoming that plague--snoring!

BIBLIOGRAPHY

Boulware, Marcus H., Ph.D., <u>Snoring: New Answers to an Old Problem.</u> American Faculty Press: Rockaway, N.J. First printing, 1974.

Brody, Jane, <u>Jane Brody's The New York Times Guide to Personal Health</u>. TIMES BOOKS, a division of Quadrangle/The New York Times Book Co., Inc.: Three Park Avenue, New York, N.Y. 10016. Seventh copyright, 1982.

Burt, John, Ed.D., and Miller, Benjamin, M.D., <u>Personal Health Behavior in Today's Society</u>. W.B. Saunders Company: Philadelphia, Pa. First printing, 1972.

Editors of <u>Prevention</u> Magazine Health Books, <u>Future Youth: How To Reverse the Aging Process</u>. Rodale Press: Emmaus, Pennsylvania. First printing, 1987.

Feltman, John, <u>Prevention's Giant Book of Health Facts</u>. Rodale Press: Emmaus, Pennsylvania. First printing, 1991.

Hensel, Bruce, M.D., <u>Smart Medicine: How to Get the Most Out of Your Medical Checkup and Stay Healthy.</u> G.P. Putnam's Sons: New York. First printing, 1989.

Jensen, Bernard, Nutritionist, <u>Nature Has a Remedy: (It Can Be Physical, Mental or Spiritual)</u>. Unity Press: P.O. Box 1037, Santa Cruz, CA 95061. First printing, 1978.

Lipman, Derek S., M.D., <u>Stop Your Husband From Snoring: A Medically Proven Program to Cure the Night's Worst Nuisance.</u> Rodale Press: Emmaus, Pennsylvania. First printing, 1990.

Morris, William, <u>The American Heritage Dictionary of the English Language.</u> Houghton Mifflin Company: Boston, Massachusetts. Seventh Edition, 1978.

Mosley, James L., <u>Snore No More!</u> International Scene Publications and Distribution Company: 34208 Aurora Rd. Suite 165, Cleveland, OH. 44139, 1990.

Rosenfeld, Dr. Isadore, M.D., <u>Modern Prevention: The New Medicine</u>. The Linden Press/ Simon and Schuster: New York. First printing, 1986.

World Book, Inc., <u>The World Book Encyclopedia</u>. World Book, Inc., a Scott Fetzer company: Chicago, IL. Copyright, 1983.

INDEX